THE
Smoothie Plan

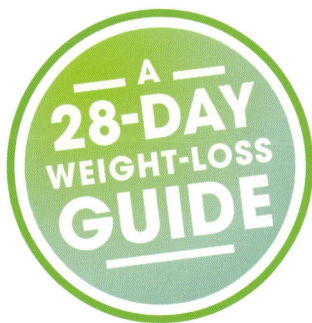

— A —
28-DAY
WEIGHT-LOSS
GUIDE

Prevention

Table of

Contents

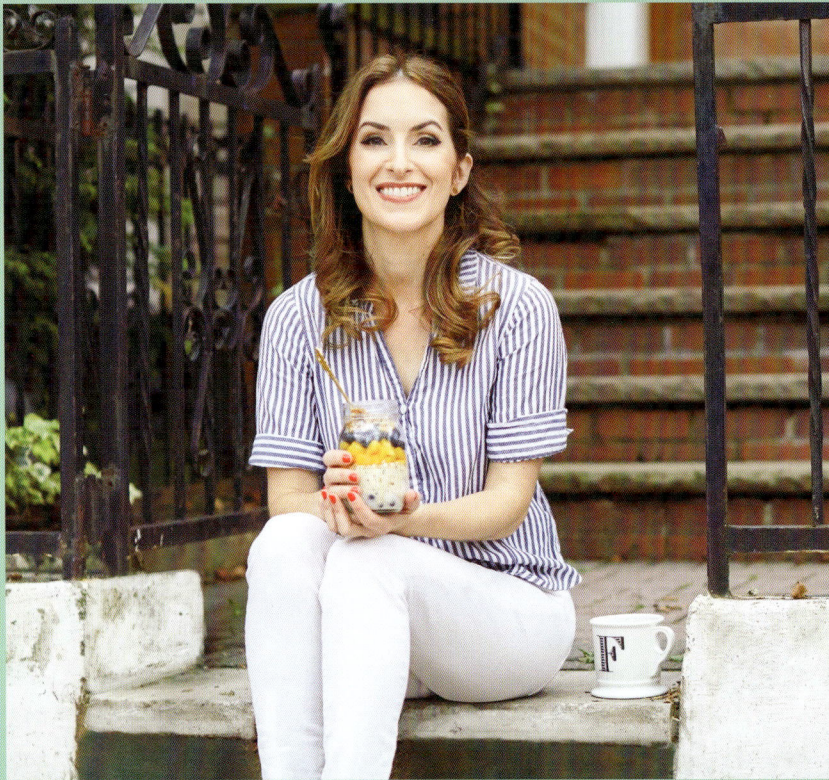

AUTHOR

Frances Largeman-Roth is a registered dietitian nutritionist, a *New York Times* best-selling author and nationally recognized nutrition and wellness expert. Frances is the author of *Feed the Belly: The Pregnant Mom's Healthy Eating Guide, Eating in Color,* and *Prevention Smoothies & Juices: 100+ Delicious Recipes for Optimal Wellness.* She is also the co-author of the bestselling *The CarbLovers Diet.*

Frances is a contributor to several publications, including *Today.com, Parents, Parade,* and *MindBodyGreen.* She has appeared on numerous national TV shows, including *The Today Show, The Dr. Oz Show, The Rachael Ray Show, Good Morning America,* and *Access Hollywood Live,* as well as QVC and CNN. Frances contributes expert quotes to national publications and helps healthy food brands share their message. She is a member of the James Beard Foundation and the Academy of Nutrition and Dietetics. She received her undergraduate degree at Cornell University and completed her dietetic internship at Columbia.

Frances is a proponent of a balanced, plant-forward lifestyle and loves helping people make healthy eating fun. Frances, her husband, and three kids live in Westchester County, NY. To learn more, visit her website: **franceslargemanroth.com.**

Intro

After more than 20 years of working with women to help them achieve healthy, balanced lifestyles through nutrition, I've learned a lot about which plans will work and which ones will fail. Probably the biggest lesson I've taken away from my experiences is that if a plan isn't easy to incorporate into your busy lifestyle, it just won't work. No one has time to make complicated recipes or fit in two-hour workouts each day. And just because your friend or a celebrity says she had great results on a plan, that doesn't mean it will work for you.

We know there are hundreds of weight loss plans out there, all claiming that they're the best way to get healthy. It's all this confusion that can make it so daunting to find a plan that will work for you. That's why smoothies are an ideal tool to help you lose weight. Nothing could be simpler than throwing ingredients (the right ones, of course!) into a blender. You'll be enjoying a smoothie for breakfast or lunch each day, and then making simple and delicious meals to round out the rest of your menus. And because we know how important it is to keep your energy levels up, we've also included plenty of healthy snack options.

Not only can smoothies help you on your weight loss journey, they're also an excellent way to increase your daily fruit and vegetable consumption. Most of us don't get enough produce in our diets, and smoothies are a fun and delicious way to get more in. Even better, those tasty fruits and vegetables contain health-boosting nutrients, plus fiber, which we know is essential for a balanced gut and a healthy weight.

BY FRANCES LARGEMAN-ROTH, R.D.N.

What are you waiting for? Grab your blender and let's go!

→

CHAPTER 1

The Basics

Smoothies vs. Juices

I'm often asked what the difference is between a smoothie and a juice, and whether one is healthier than the other. The truth is that they can both be incredibly good for you. But when it comes to weight loss, smoothies are the clear winner. Why? It's all about the F-word—FIBER! Fiber is your friend when it comes to feeling full and satisfied. And when you juice a fruit or vegetable, you're removing most of the fiber. Smoothies, on the other hand, retain all of the filling fiber, and make it much easier to eat more fruits and vegetables every day.

ANATOMY OF A SMOOTHIE

Over the years clients have complained to me that their smoothies never turn out the way they want them to. Sometimes they're too thick, or sometimes their blender gets jammed up, leaving them frustrated and hungry—argh! It turns out that there's a right—and a wrong—way to add smoothie ingredients to your blender. In addition to our steps below, always check the manufacturer's directions before using your blender for the first time.

STEP 1:

Add your liquid first. This includes water, juice, yogurt, and milk or plant milk. The liquid in the bottom will help to create a vortex, which will make it easier for the other ingredients to be incorporated into the smoothie mixture.

STEP 2:

Add in nut or seed butters, nuts, spices, protein powders, dates, sweeteners, and any other add-ins. You want these ingredients to be evenly distributed throughout your smoothie. No one wants a big slurp full of protein powder!

STEP 3:

Add your fruits and veggies. If using all frozen items, you may run into issues with the blade jamming up. It's ideal to use a combo of fresh and frozen items, if possible. When most of your ingredients are frozen, add half of the frozen ones, blend, then add the rest.

STEP 4:

If you're using ice, add it now.

STEP 5:

Blend until creamy. If the mixture is too thick, add additional water. If items are getting stuck, turn off the blender and use a spatula to push them down and away from the blades. Blend again, pour into a glass and enjoy!

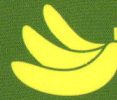

Freezing Bananas

Lots of our recipes call for a banana, oftentimes frozen. Bananas are the quintessential smoothie ingredient because they not only add subtle sweetness to your smoothie and give your blend lots of body, they also provide potassium for your muscles. Using frozen bananas is a smart way to make your smoothie thicker and it also keeps the fruit from turning brown on you. Here's the right way to freeze them:

1

Start with ripe, but not mushy, bananas. The peel should be yellow, with just a little bit of green at the ends.

2

Line a baking sheet with parchment and set aside.

3

Peel the bananas, then slice them into rounds and place in a single layer on the prepared baking sheet.

4

Freeze for 2 hours, until solid.

5

Transfer the frozen rounds to a resealable plastic freezer bag for up to six months.

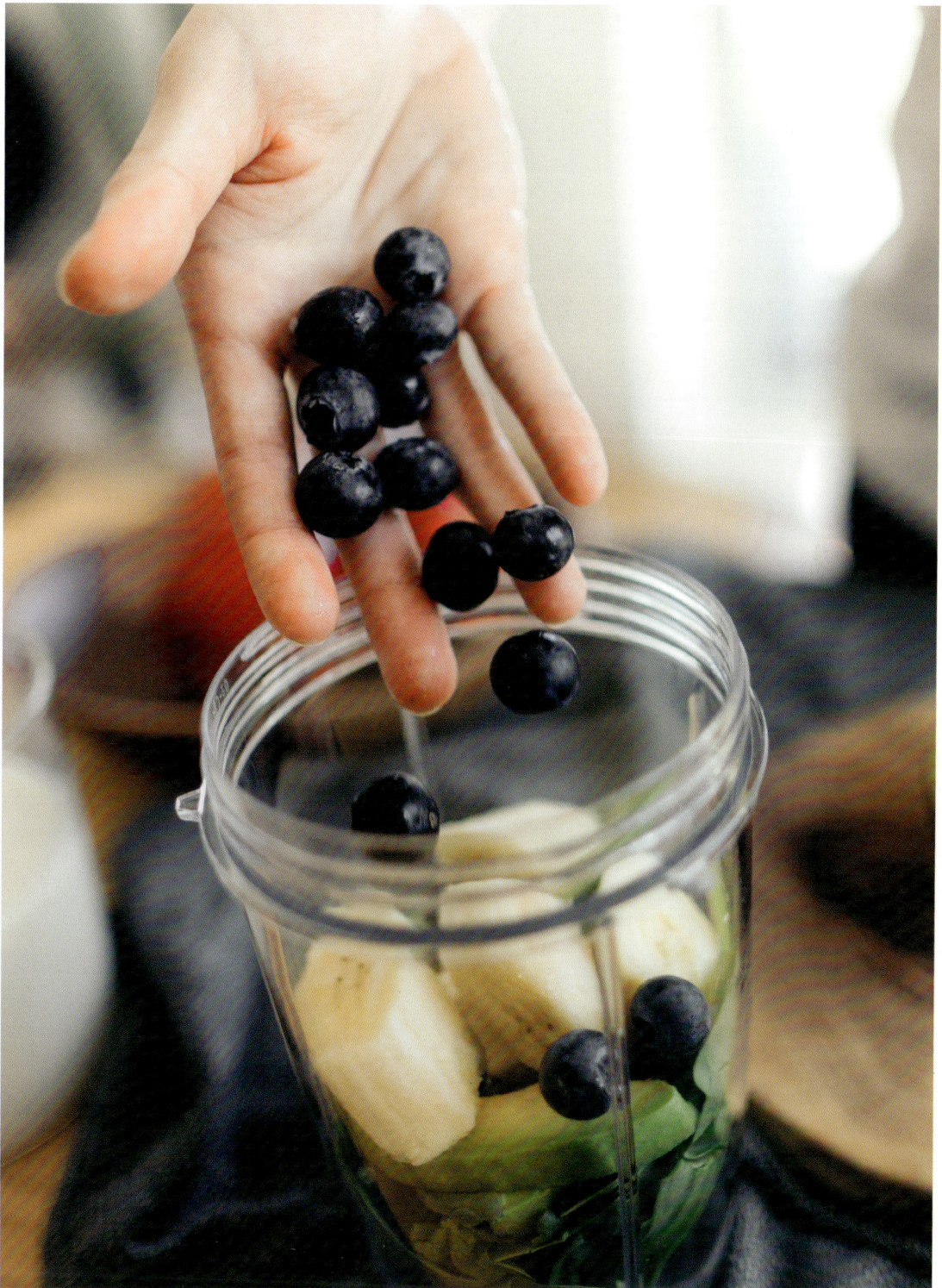

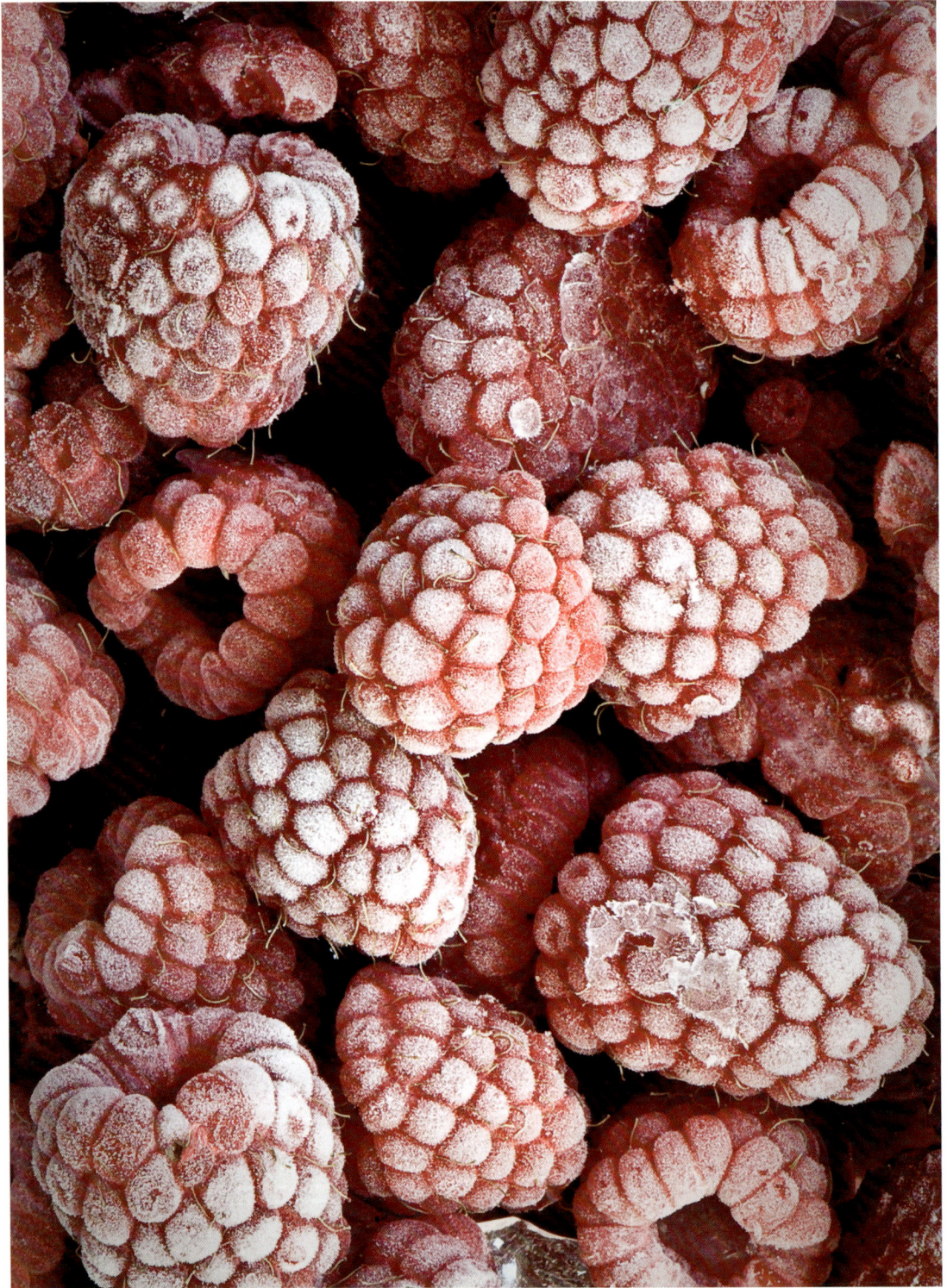

IDEAL INGREDIENTS

When it comes to versatility, smoothies win—hands down. You can blend up virtually any fruit and most veggies and add in basically any combination of other ingredients that taste good to you. Of course, we think that certain blends are more delicious and nutritious than others.

Frozen vs. Fresh

Lots of people wonder if they need to use all fresh produce to get the most nutrients from their smoothie. The answer is a definite NO! Frozen fruits and vegetables are an excellent choice for smoothies. Frozen fruits and veggies are picked at the peak of ripeness and then flash frozen, which seals in nutrients. And the best part about frozen produce is that there's literally no waste! You can use what you need and then return the rest to the freezer.

Bags of berries, pineapple, mango, sliced peaches, and more are wonderful to keep on hand in the freezer. They're incredibly cost effective too, especially if you like to use organic produce. You can also save produce that you know you won't use up in time by freezing it. You can literally freeze almost anything! Just be sure to wash and then thoroughly dry (that's super important) your produce before transferring it to a resealable zip-top freezer bag. You can keep your frozen goodies for up to 6 months, so write the date on the bag.

Seasonal Ingredients

I think of seasonal ingredients as accessories. They help add variety to your smoothie repertoire, just like a new necklace can make a favorite LBD feel fresh again. Plus, in-season fruits and veggies are super nutritious. Those ripe berries and peaches don't last very long, so either use them up quickly or cut them up and store them in an airtight container in the freezer. And wash ripe produce just before using to prevent it from getting moldy.

Year-Round Ingredients

These are the staples that you'll be grabbing over and over again to make healthy smoothies. Bananas may be a tropical fruit, but you'll find them all year. Baby spinach, shredded carrots, chopped kale, avocados, and ginger root are other ingredients that work well in smoothies, no matter what season it is.

If you don't have any issues digesting lactose and enjoy milk, feel free to use it in your smoothies. It's a fantastic source of protein, calcium, and potassium, as well as vitamins A and D. But if you prefer to use plant milks, we recommend keeping several types in your fridge. We like using different plant milks for different types of smoothies. When we want to add more body, oat milk works best. To balance out the bitterness of greens and spices like turmeric, coconut milk is often the best choice. What's nice about many of the plant-based milks is that they come in shelf-stable packaging, so you don't need to refrigerate them until you've opened them.

Freezing Berries

Enjoy the flavors of summer berries year-round by buying extra when they're in season and freezing them. Here's how to do it:

1 Rinse the berries gently with running water.

2 If freezing strawberries, remove the hull with a paring knife or huller.

3 Completely dry the berries. Spread them out on a clean kitchen towel or pat them dry.

4 Line a baking sheet with parchment paper. Spread the dry berries in a single layer on the baking sheet.

5 Place the baking sheet in the freezer until berries are completely frozen, about 2 to 3 hours.

6 Transfer frozen berries to resealable zip-top freezer bags, add a label, and store in the freezer.

7 Use in your favorite smoothie!

CHAPTER 2

Smoothies and Weight Loss

How Smoothies Help with Weight Loss

Anyone who has tried to lose weight or maintain a healthy weight knows that the more complicated a plan is, the harder it will be to follow. Plans that call for hard-to-find ingredients and time-consuming recipes are just too much work. We're pretty sure you have more important (and fun!) things to do with your time.

Smoothies, on the other hand, are about the easiest thing you can make in the kitchen. They require absolutely no cooking and are ready in just minutes. It's quick and easy to clean up after smoothie prep. Plus, you'll feel energized and satisfied after sipping our smoothies, which means you'll want to come back for more.

Is a Smoothie Really Healthy?

You may have read something on the Internet about smoothies NOT being the key to weight loss. Many people think that smoothies are loaded with sugar. It's true that a smoothie that you buy in a shop could have added sugars from syrups and sweeteners, and we should all be cutting back on the amount of added sugars in our diets for overall health. But a smoothie that you make at home can be incredibly healthy. Fruits and some vegetables do contain natural sugars, which is what makes them taste so delicious. But you don't need to avoid natural sugars. The naturally occurring sugars in berries, bananas, and apples are a fantastic energy source! And—this is important—the natural sugars in fruits and vegetables come along with fiber and important health-boosting nutrients, which make a complete nutrient package.

And the truth is that most Americans—in fact 9 out of 10 of us—just aren't getting enough fruits and vegetables. According to the Centers for Disease Control and Prevention (CDC), eating a diet rich in fruits and veggies daily can help reduce the risk of many chronic diseases, including type 2 diabetes, heart disease, certain cancers, and obesity. So, boosting your plant intake with daily smoothies can not only help keep you healthy, but also trim.

The power of smoothies is that you can create a balanced, satisfying, and budget-friendly meal in minutes. You can fit in a serving of fruit and a serving of veggies (even kale!), 15 to 20 grams of protein, and 10-plus grams of fiber into a delicious drink that you can take on the go. That's something that is nearly impossible to achieve with any other type of meal. What's more, you can add functional ingredients, like inflammation-fighting turmeric and heart-smart chia seeds, to your blends without having to cook a thing.

We think smoothies are pretty amazing, and we're convinced you'll be a convert too. But a diet made entirely of smoothies wouldn't be balanced long-term, and you'd probably miss having more texture in your food. That's why we've paired our smoothies with delicious meals that are both satisfying and designed to help you achieve your healthy weight goals. No deprivation here!

How to Make a Balanced Smoothie

There's an art and science behind making a balanced and satisfying smoothie. You can't simply dump a bunch of ingredients into your blender and hope for the best. Feeling satisfied is the key to a smoothie that will help you lose weight, and there are certain ingredients that will keep you feeling fuller than others. Let's take a look at how to build the perfect smoothie. Your smoothies should have these three elements: fiber, fat, and protein.

Not only do fiber, healthy fats, and protein help you feel satisfied so that you're not reaching for unhealthy snacks, the combination of these nutrients also helps keep your blood sugar steady, so that you can avoid spikes and dips in energy. That means you'll have consistent energy to do the things you love!

What Goes In a Great Smoothie

FIBER

You've heard it before—fiber helps you feel full. But just like we're not eating enough fruits and veggies, we're also not getting enough fiber in our diets. The United States Department of Agriculture's (USDA) Dietary Guidelines recommends getting between 25 and 38 grams of fiber daily. On average, though, most of us only get 16g daily. Smoothies can help us boost our fiber intake and reach our goals, which is helpful not only for getting to a healthy weight, but also for our overall wellness.

High-fiber foods include fruit, leafy greens, nuts, seeds, and whole grains—all of which are featured in our healthy smoothies!

HEALTHY FAT

If you survived the fat-phobic '90s, you remember a time when all types of fat were something to flee from and were synonymous with weight gain. Thankfully, the time to embrace fat and all that it can do for you has arrived. Humans need fat for so many reasons—it helps us absorb certain vitamins and is involved with the creation of important hormones in the body. It's also what helps us feel satisfied after a meal. Without fat, we're often left wanting more after we've eaten.

There are fats we should avoid and cut back on. It's smart to skip sources of trans fat, and to watch your intake of saturated fat, which primarily comes from animal sources, like meat and cheese. The good fats to include are monounsaturated and polyunsaturated fats. Monounsaturated fats are found in nuts, nut butter, avocados, seeds, olive oil, and other plant oils. Polyunsaturated fat sources include soybean, corn and sunflower oil, as well as fatty fish, walnuts, and flax seeds.

Our smoothies include healthy fat from avocado, nuts, nut milk and nut butters, chia, hemp, and flax seeds.

PROTEIN

This nutrient is key for building and maintaining muscle—which naturally declines as we age. Protein has also been shown in several studies to help with satiety—the feeling of being full. Getting enough protein can help us lose weight while preserving our muscles. For people who have lost weight and regained it, protein has been shown to be helpful in reducing the amount of weight regained over time.

I always recommend getting 1 gram of protein per kilogram of body weight. You can easily calculate that by taking your weight in pounds and dividing the result by 2.2 to get kilograms. For example, a 150-pound person should be getting approximately 68g of protein each day.

While protein is important for weight loss, more isn't necessarily better. Our bodies can only utilize 30 grams at a time. So, bulking up your smoothie with more than that would only be adding extra calories to your shake.

Our smoothies are protein-packed thanks to the inclusion of nuts, seeds, yogurt, and protein powder. Some smoothies have plenty of protein from dairy and nuts, but others need more to provide the satiety that you need to feel full. That's where we've added in a scoop or half a scoop of protein powder to boost the protein content and deliver a smoothie that's nutritionally balanced.

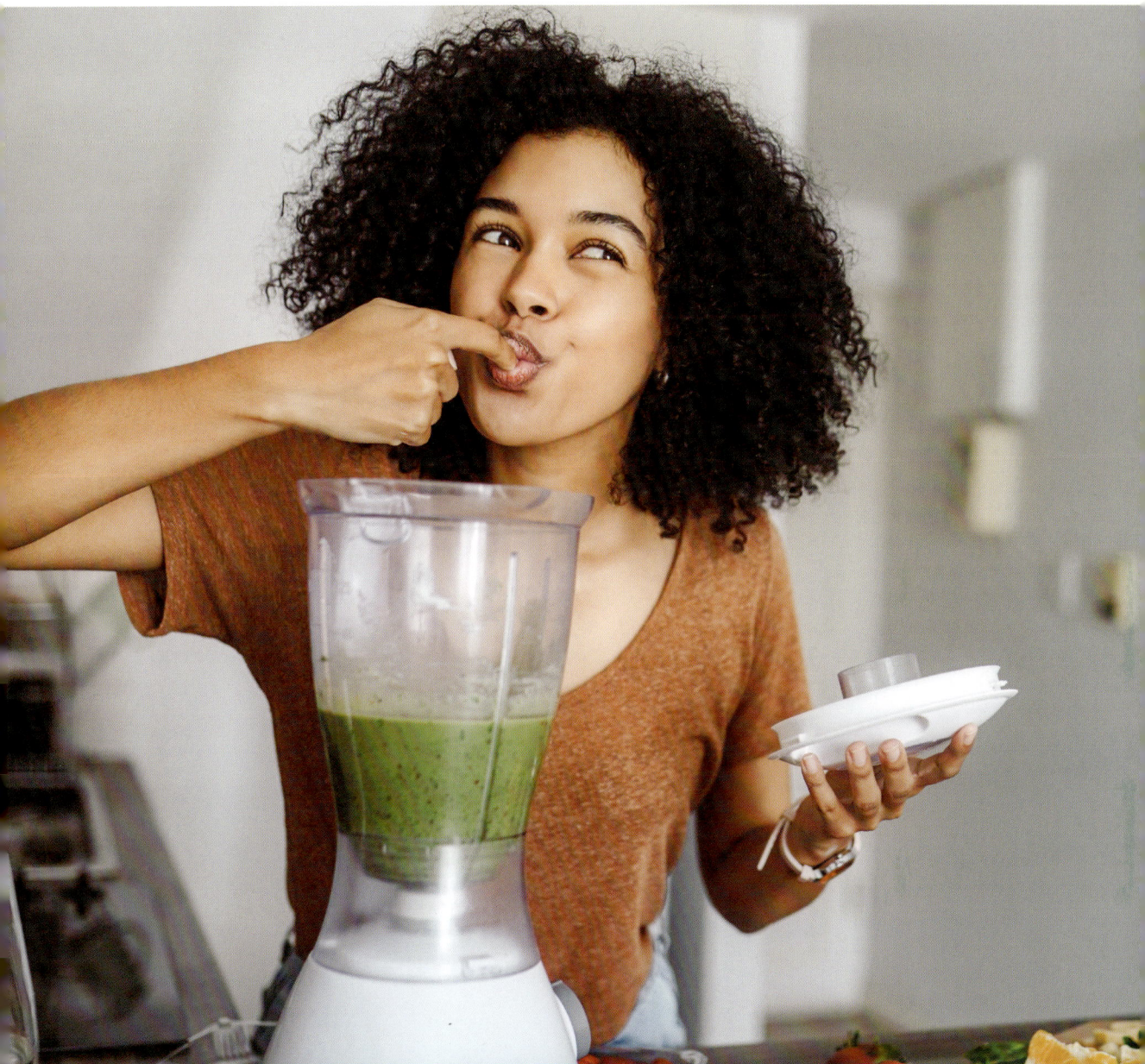

→ How to Clean Your Blender

Blenders can be tough to clean if you let them sit too long—yuck! Here's the trick to easy clean-up. After pouring your smoothie into a glass, immediately add warm water to the blender jar until it's about ¾ of the way full. Squeeze in a couple of drops of liquid dish soap, put the cover back on, and blend. Your blender will be spotless in about 30 seconds. Give it a rinse and let it air dry until next time.

PROTEIN POWDERS

Protein powders are an efficient and convenient way to make sure that you're getting enough protein in your diet. A scoop of protein powder will deliver between 15 and 20g of protein and will provide anywhere from 90 to 200 calories. There are a ton of protein powders on the market these days from various sources. The options can be dizzying! If possible, we recommend trying a packet or two of various kinds before committing to a large container, since protein powders can be expensive.

When shopping for protein powders, be sure to take a minute or two to read the ingredient list. Avoid those with added and artificial sweeteners. And if you're sensitive to gluten, make sure the label says that the product is gluten-free. If you know you're sensitive to added fibers, skip powders with psyllium fiber or coconut husk fiber as they may make you gassy and cause bloating.

Our smoothie recipes may use a few types of protein powders, but you don't need to purchase all the powders! Find one that you like, and rest assured that you can use it in all the different smoothies. Here's a breakdown of the most popular types:

WHEY

This is the gold standard. Whey is a by-product of the cheese-making process and contains all 9 essential amino acids, which are the building blocks of protein. When combined with strength training, such as lifting weights, it has been shown to help build muscle. Whey contains lactose, a sugar in milk, so it's not for anyone who is sensitive to lactose.

SOY

Shown to be as effective at building muscle as whey protein, this plant-based protein is very popular. Soy also contains isoflavones, which have been shown to protect against heart disease, osteoporosis, and some cancers. Soy is a known allergen, though, so if you need to avoid it, be sure to skip powders with this ingredient.

PEA

A vegan alternative, this eco-friendly powder works well in flavor-packed smoothies but may taste a little grassy in more delicately flavored recipes.

BROWN RICE

This easy-to-digest protein works well in both smoothies and baked goods. Since it doesn't have all the essential amino acids, you'll want to alternate it with another type of protein powder.

HEMP

This powder is made from high-fiber hemp seeds and packs omega-3 and -6 fats, as well as protein. Since it contains fat, hemp protein should be refrigerated to keep it fresh.

ALMOND

Almond protein powder is made from just almonds. You can use almond protein powder in your smoothies, as well as in baking, and it also delivers on calcium and potassium.

PLANT BLENDS

You'll find various plant blends on the market. These combine pea protein with various other ingredients, like sprouted grains, alfalfa, brown rice protein, or algae. Blends can be good because they provide protein from a variety of sources.

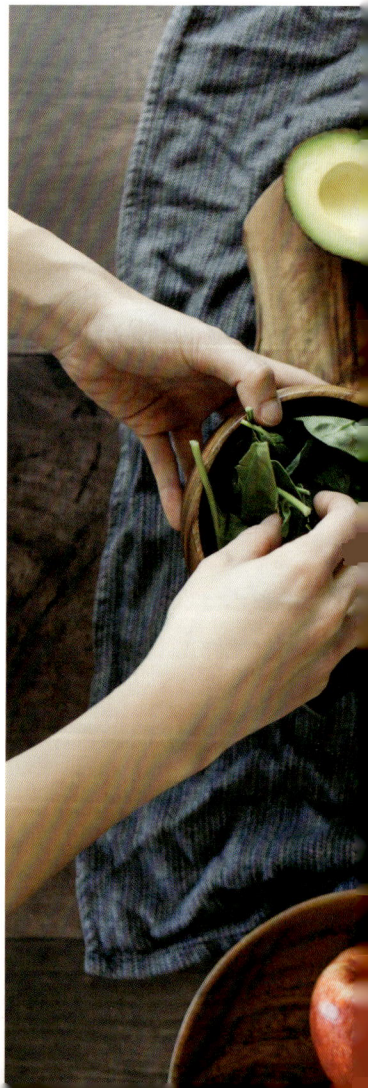

Smoothie Dos & Don'ts

One of the things we love about smoothies is how versatile they are. You can use your favorite ingredients to create blends that satisfy your personal taste preferences and cravings. But as with most things, you can certainly overdo it on some ingredients. Here are some basic dos and don'ts to keep in mind when crafting smoothies to help you lose weight:

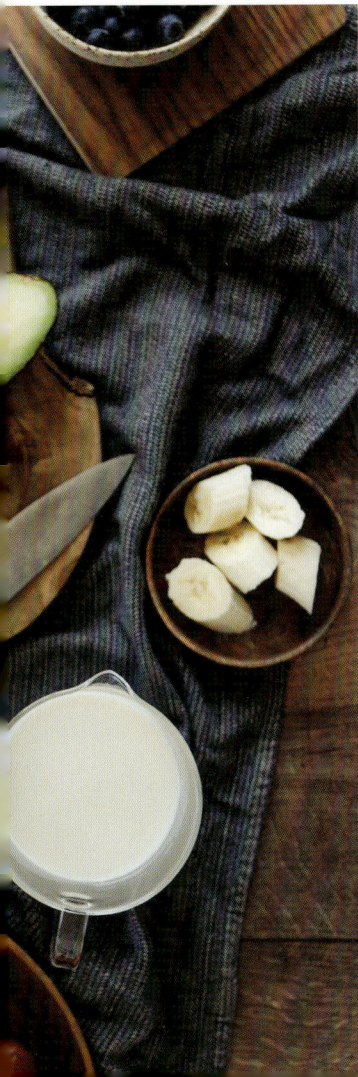

DO'S:

Experiment!: We know you'll find a favorite smoothie in this book that you'll go back to over and over again. That's great, but it's also fun to experiment with different fruits, veggies, nut butters, and more.

Remember your ratios: While pretty much anything will mix up in your blender, you do need an appropriate amount of liquid to keep things flowing. So, feel free to replace almond milk with oat milk, or hemp seeds with flax seeds—just keep the amounts the same.

Prep like a pro: Most smoothies come together so quickly that you really don't need to do much prep. But as with many things in life,

a little prep goes a long way. We like making smoothie prep packs to make our smoothie sessions even faster. You simply gather all the dry ingredients for your smoothie, place them in a resealable plastic bag or reusable silicone bag, and place it in the freezer. Then when you're ready to blend, place your liquid in the bottom of your blender, pour in the contents of your smoothie pack, and blend!

DON'TS:

Oversweeten: You'll notice that we haven't added much extra sweetness to our smoothies. A touch of honey or pure maple syrup is a great way to make your smoothie taste delicious, but you don't want to add so much that it becomes more like a dessert. If adding additional sweetness beyond what the recipe calls for, make sure to use a measuring spoon and start with a ½ teaspoon, which will only add 10 calories. Add more if you need it, but keep in mind that a tablespoon will add an extra 60 calories to your smoothie. Try to keep added sugars to no more than a teaspoon.

Overload your blender: You may have some items in your fridge that you want to use up, but consider how much to add before you hit the "on" button on your blender. We are all for reducing food waste, but packing too much stuff into your blender at once can be a recipe for a blender that gets locked up, or a smoothie that's just too thick to drink.

Be too virtuous: Some people think that if 1 cup of spinach or baby kale is good, 3 cups are better. While smoothies are a great way to fit in more veggies, if you add too much of a good thing, you may end up with a smoothie that is too bitter to enjoy. And you may be tempted to omit an ingredient to lower the calories in a smoothie, but please fight the urge! Drinking a smoothie that has too few calories won't keep you full, and that may have you visiting the snack machine before lunch.

CHAPTER 3

The Meal Plan

Getting Started

We've created a 28-day meal plan to help you feel energized and satisfied while you lose weight. The plan includes plenty of variety, but if simplicity works better for you, just pick one or two smoothies, lunches, and dinners and keep them in rotation during the week.

The meal plan is designed to supply you with 1,500 to 1,600 calories per day, which should help you lose up to 1 pound per week, depending on your activity level. The recipes we chose have a good balance of calories, fiber, protein, and fat to help you feel full and satisfied. And we've evenly distributed calories throughout the day so that you'll never feel hungry or deprived. Certain smoothies have enough calories on their own, while we've paired others with a side, such as avocado toast or a hard-boiled egg, to make sure you have plenty of fuel to keep you feeling great.

You can start the plan on any day of the week you'd like! Doing your grocery shopping before the day you'd like to begin will help to set you up for success. You can also familiarize yourself with the ingredients in the recipes and decide which meals you're going to make. We want this plan to work for YOU, so don't worry about making every single recipe! Prioritize the smoothies, and then make as many of the meals as you have time for.

WHEN TO DRINK YOUR SMOOTHIE

We've included a smoothie for breakfast on most days, but have used them for lunch on some days to help highlight that you can use them when they work best for you. If you want to have a smoothie for lunch every day, that works too! Simply use one of the non-smoothie breakfast recipes, like Oatmeal with Cranberries and Pecans (p. 107), as your breakfast.

WHAT ELSE TO EAT ON THE PLAN

Most lunch and dinner recipes are used twice within the same week. You'll see that some of our lunch and dinner recipes make four servings. If you have a friend or family member who would like to follow the plan along with you, you can split the servings with them. If not, we recommend either freezing the leftovers to save time the following week, or halving the recipe if that's easier. Just note that you'll need to buy less of the ingredients on the shopping list.

Day 1 of each week is designed as a Meatless Monday. If that's the eating style you prefer, you can find other vegan and vegetarian recipes by looking for the VEGAN or VEGETARIAN label next to the recipes.

Smoothies and dishes with at least 5 grams of fiber have the HIGH FIBER tag, and ones with at least 15 grams of protein are labeled PROTEIN-PACKED.

We've included one snack each day on the plan. You can use this whenever you'd like! I would recommend having it either mid-morning or mid-afternoon. You can pick a snack from any day of the week. All are healthy and balanced and provide energy without a crash. Also, if you still feel hungry after dinner, you can always enjoy a piece of fruit in the evening.

CUSTOMIZE YOUR SMOOTHIE

You can add a scoop of unflavored protein powder to pretty much any smoothie recipe. Vanilla protein powder works well with berries and most other fruits, while chocolate blends up nicely with nut butters, cocoa powder, coffee, and banana. If you see a smoothie recipe in the plan that doesn't include protein powder, feel free to add a scoop. Just keep in mind that you may need to add a little more water or milk for it to blend up perfectly.

Hate protein powders? That's fine too! We get it— they're not for everyone. If you plan to skip them, just make sure that you're including high-protein snacks each day, like nuts, Greek yogurt, and cheese. Also, you can use unsweetened nut butters instead of protein powder in your smoothie, but they will add more calories and not as much protein per serving (about 7g of protein and 190 calories per 2-tablespoon serving). Another great ingredient to try is peanut butter powder, which gives you 6g of protein per 2 tablespoons, for just 60 calories.

Whatever you do—don't skimp on protein. It not only helps you feel satisfied, but it's also essential for maintaining muscle. And a body with more muscle burns more calories!

After the 28 Days

We've included a selection of our favorite smoothies in the meal plan, but you'll find tons more on pages 122 to 174. You get smoothie recipes that have varying calorie amounts so you're guaranteed to enjoy a delicious and nutritionally balanced option whether you feel like having it as a low-calorie snack or as a filling meal. A hard-boiled egg (70 calories) or a piece of avocado or almond toast (260 calories) can round out your meal nicely. And if the smoothie you're making has less than 10 grams of protein per serving, you can boost it by adding a scoop of protein powder (about 160 calories).

We hope you'll love the smoothie recipes, as well as the other recipes in the book, and will continue to use them to support your wellness. While it can sometimes be time-consuming, preparing your own meals and snacks is always the healthiest way to go.

Using the Wellness Tracker

We know you're busy! And we want you to succeed on this plan, so we've included Wellness Trackers to help you stay on top of your physical and emotional health during all 28 days. The Wellness Tracker will help you quickly document how you feel after each meal. Did you feel full after breakfast or were you still hungry? Maybe you liked a few lunch recipes a lot but didn't care for others. Tracking how you feel after a meal can help you pinpoint areas that you need to focus on. For example, maybe you didn't sleep well last night and today you're noticing that you're craving sweets. It's helpful to keep in mind that many different factors affect your appetite and mood. The more we can tune into how food affects us, the better equipped we'll be to handle what life throws at us—even on Mondays!

Ready, Set, Prep!

Some folks feel best when they can prep the ingredients for as many meals as possible, while others would rather make each meal as they need it. Both ways can work—you just need to figure out what works best with your individual schedule and lifestyle.

We recommended prepping a little bit on Sunday—or the day before you plan to start the plan. It can be as simple as chopping some veggies and washing fruit, or as extensive as making recipes from start to finish. You can even prep something as simple as a smoothie.

If you want to prep your smoothies in advance, we recommend getting a personal blender. This style has a cup that attaches directly to the base, and it often allows you to drink directly from the cup. You can use the cup to prepare all your smoothie ingredients in advance—for example, you can prep a breakfast smoothie the night before a busy morning. Put your ingredients in the blender cup, cover it, and place it in the fridge. Then the next morning, just roll out of bed, blend, and go!

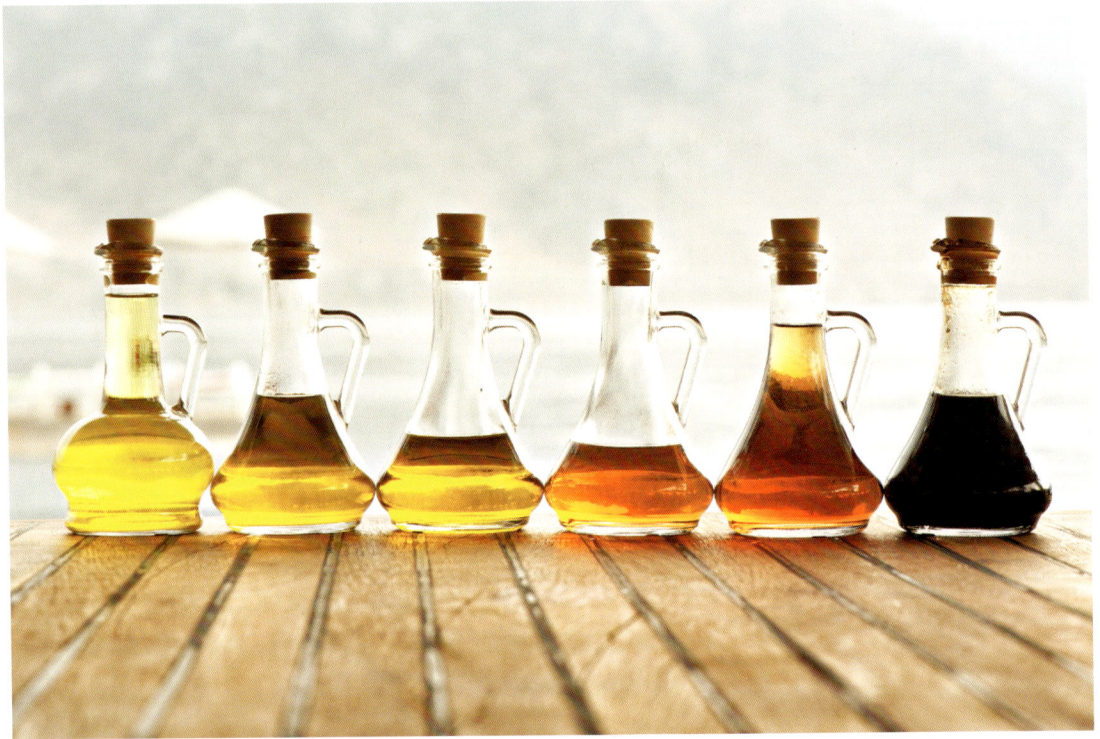

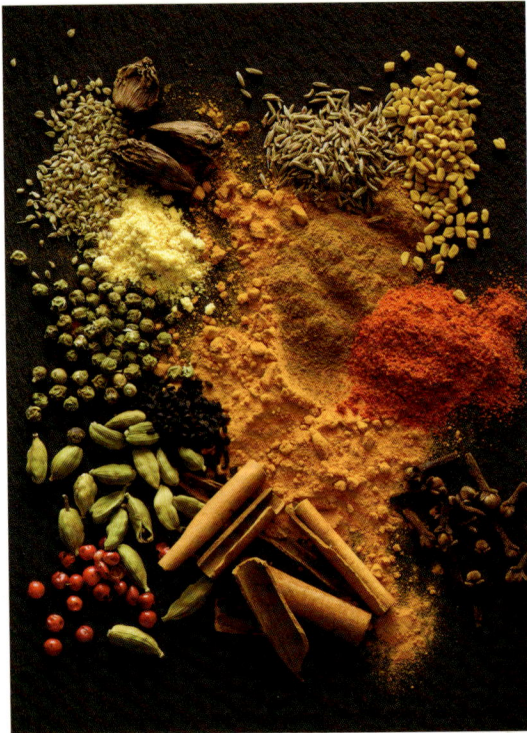

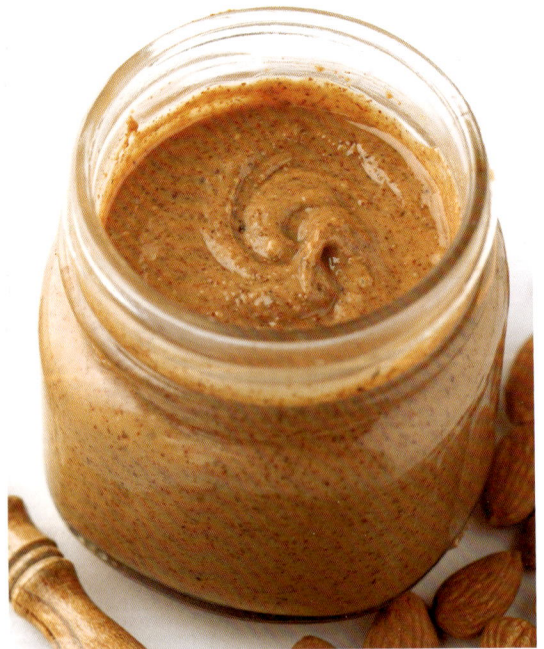

Here are some ideas for prepping meal and snack ingredients:

1 Many of our smoothies call for ice, so fill up those ice cube trays!

2 Wash and chop veggies like kale, cauliflower, and broccoli.

3 Pre-rinse garbanzo beans so that they're ready to be used.

4 Make grains ahead of time, then just reheat for serving.

5 Measure out nuts for snacks and package them in to-go containers.

6 Cut up melon and wash grapes.

7 Cook proteins in advance, then portion and refrigerate or freeze till you need them.

8 Use frozen fruit and veggies whenever possible. They're already washed and chopped!

9 If you're using fresh produce for smoothies, place them in the freezer ahead of time so they're nice and chilled when it's time to throw them in your blender.

10 Hard-boil eggs and park them in the fridge so they're ready to eat when breakfast calls for it.

Pantry Staples

Before you dive in, figure out what'll make this plan easier for you to follow. Do you want to follow the weekly plan exactly, or mix it up? Do you have some of the ingredients on hand already? Here's a list of pantry staples you'll need to have on hand to complete the plan.

1 bottle red wine vinegar

1 small bottle apple cider vinegar

1 small bottle less-sodium soy sauce

1 small bottle rice vinegar

1 16-oz bottle olive oil, preferably extra virgin

1 small bottle vegetable oil

1 small bottle canola oil

1 small jar honey

1 16-oz jar almond butter

1 small jar creamy peanut butter

1 small bottle pure maple syrup

1 small package brown sugar

1 small jar ground cayenne pepper

1 small jar crushed red pepper

1 small jar chili powder

1 small jar ground cumin

1 small jar ground turmeric

1 small jar ground ginger

1 small jar ground coriander

1 small jar dried oregano

1 small jar ground cinnamon

1 small jar red pepper flakes

1 small container cornmeal

1 small pouch ground flaxseed

1 small pouch hulled hemp seeds

1 small pouch chia seeds

1 container protein powder, either whey- or plant-based

1 container vanilla whey protein powder

Kosher salt

Black pepper

Week 1

Shopping List

PRODUCE

3 large avocados

1 5-oz bag baby arugula

1 small package baby carrots

1 small package shredded carrots

6 medium bananas

1 small bunch cilantro

4 cups cubed melon

1 seedless cucumber

3 Persian cucumbers

1 small bunch flat-leaf parsley

1 small piece fresh ginger (about 1½ in.)

1 lemon

1 lime

1 sprig oregano

1 48-oz bag frozen pineapple chunks

½ small pineapple

1 10-oz bag frozen shelled edamame

1 small container grape tomatoes

½ lb mixed cherry, grape, and campari tomatoes

1 small container strawberries

1 16-oz bag kale

1 large scallion

½ medium head (about 1 lb) cauliflower

1 8-oz package pitted dates

3 small red onions

1 8-oz package snow peas

1 bunch upland watercress

DAIRY & REFRIGERATED

1 small container feta cheese

½ dozen eggs

4 oz Gruyère cheese

1 lb pizza dough

1 32-oz container plain Greek yogurt

1 32-oz container unsweetened almond milk

1 10-oz container hummus

1 12-oz container coconut water

MEATS & PROTEINS

2 14-oz blocks extra-firm tofu

1 lb large shrimp

1 6-oz can salmon

PANTRY

1 small jar pitted Kalamata olives

1 peanut butter squeeze pack

2 oz (about 46 pieces) almonds

1 15-oz can chickpeas

1 small jar capers

1 small package confectioners' sugar

1 8-oz box rotini (spiral) pasta

1 box wild rice

1 small container cornmeal

1 small container cornstarch

1 small jar curry powder

1 small bar dark chocolate, optional

1 small container miso paste

1 oz shelled pistachios

1 small package quinoa

1 small bag roasted cashews

1 small jar sesame seeds

1 7-oz bottle Thai sweet chili sauce

1 5-oz bottle toasted sesame oil

1 8-oz container unsweetened cocoa powder

1 loaf whole-grain bread (look for whole grains as the first ingredient)

Meal Plan

Day 1

BREAKFAST
Creamy Kale
Smoothie (p. 62)

LUNCH
Chickpea Pasta Salad
in a Jar (p. 79)

DINNER
Crispy Tofu Bowl
(p. 81; 1 serving)

SNACK
1 oz almonds +
1 medium banana

Day 2

BREAKFAST
Sweet 'n' Spicy Tropical
Smoothie (p. 63) +
1 piece almond butter
toast (p. 27)

LUNCH
Charred Shrimp
and Avocado Salad
(p. 83; 1 serving)

DINNER
Asian Salmon Bowl
(p. 85; 1 serving)

SNACK
¼ cup hummus +
⅔ cup baby carrots

Day 3

BREAKFAST
Creamy Kale
Smoothie (p. 62) +
1 hard-boiled egg

LUNCH
LEFTOVER
Crispy Tofu Bowl

DINNER
LEFTOVER
Charred Shrimp and
Avocado Salad

SNACK
1 banana + 1 peanut
butter squeeze pack

Day 4

BREAKFAST
Curry Avocado Crispy
Egg Toast (p. 86)

LUNCH
Sweet 'n' Spicy Tropical
Smoothie (p. 63) +
1 piece almond butter
toast (p. 29)

DINNER
LEFTOVER
Asian Salmon Bowl

SNACK
2 cups cubed melon +
½ oz pistachios

Day 5

BREAKFAST
Cocoa-Almond
Smoothie (p. 65) +
1 piece avocado toast
(p. 30)

LUNCH
Crispy Tofu Bowl (p. 81)

DINNER
Roasted Cauliflower
Pizza (p. 89; 2 slices) +
Greek Salad (p. 91)

SNACK
¼ cup hummus +
⅔ cup baby carrots

Day 6

BREAKFAST
Strawberry-Avocado
Refresher (p. 64):
Boost the nutrition of
this delicious smoothie
by adding 1 scoop
of protein powder.

LUNCH
LEFTOVER Roasted
Cauliflower Pizza
(2 slices) + Greek Salad

DINNER
Charred Shrimp and
Avocado Salad (p. 83)

SNACK
2 cups cubed melon +
½ oz pistachios

Day 7

BREAKFAST
Cocoa-Almond
Smoothie (p. 65)

LUNCH
Chickpea Pasta Salad
in a Jar (p. 79)

DINNER
LEFTOVER
Charred Shrimp and
Avocado Salad

SNACK
1 oz almonds
(about 23 pieces) +
1 medium banana

Day 1

BREAKFAST
Creamy Kale
Smoothie (p. 62)

LUNCH
Chickpea Pasta Salad
in a Jar (p. 79)

DINNER
Crispy Tofu Bowl
(p. 81; 1 serving)

SNACK
1 oz almonds +
1 medium banana

NUTRITION (Per Day)
1,780 cal, 68 g pro,
207 g carb, 30 g fiber,
72 g sugars (16 g added
sugars), 79.5 g fat
(13.5 g sat fat),
1,265 mg sodium

WATER

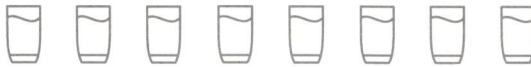

MOVEMENT/WORKOUT Y ☐ N ☐

ACTIVITY: _____
_____
_____

DURATION: _____
_____
_____

INTENSITY: _____
_____

SLEEP

Bedtime Last Night: _____ : _____

Wake Time This Morning: _____ : _____

_____
_____
_____
_____

MOOD

☺ ☺ ☹

_____
_____
_____
_____

Day 2

BREAKFAST
Sweet 'n' Spicy Tropical Smoothie (p. 63) + 1 piece almond butter toast: Spread 1 Tbsp almond butter on 1 slice whole-grain bread

LUNCH
Charred Shrimp and Avocado Salad (p. 83; 1 serving)

DINNER
Asian Salmon Bowl (p. 85; 1 serving)

SNACK
¼ cup hummus + ⅔ cup baby carrots

NUTRITION (Per Day)
1,325 cal, 65 g pro, 114 g carb, 23 g fiber, 27 g sugars (3 g sugars), 72 g fat (10 g sat fat), 2,160 mg sodium

WATER

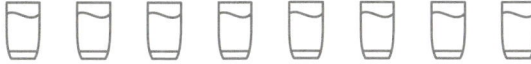

MOVEMENT/WORKOUT Y ☐ N ☐

ACTIVITY: _____
_____
_____

DURATION: _____
_____

INTENSITY: _____
_____

SLEEP

Bedtime Last Night: _____ : _____

Wake Time This Morning: _____ : _____

_____
_____
_____

MOOD

_____
_____
_____

Day 3

BREAKFAST
Creamy Kale
Smoothie (p. 62) +
1 hard-boiled egg

LUNCH
LEFTOVER
Crispy Tofu Bowl

DINNER
LEFTOVER
Charred Shrimp and
Avocado Salad

SNACK
1 banana + 1 peanut
butter squeeze pack

NUTRITION (Per Day)
1,670 cal, 76 g pro,
154 g carb, 22 g fiber,
76 g sugars (16 g added
sugars), 87. 5 g fat
(16 g sat fat), 1,560 mg
sodium

WATER

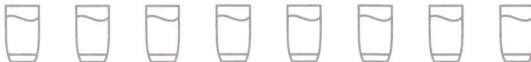

MOVEMENT/WORKOUT Y ☐ **N** ☐

ACTIVITY: _____

_____

DURATION: _____

_____

INTENSITY: _____

_____

SLEEP

Bedtime Last Night: _____ : _____

Wake Time This Morning: _____ : _____

_____

_____

_____

MOOD

☺ 😐 ☹

_____

_____

_____

Day 4

BREAKFAST
Curry Avocado Crispy Egg Toast (p. 86)

LUNCH
Sweet 'n' Spicy Tropical Smoothie (p. 63) + 1 piece almond butter toast: Spread 1 Tbsp almond butter on 1 slice whole-grain bread

DINNER
LEFTOVER
Asian Salmon Bowl

SNACK
2 cups cubed melon + ½ oz pistachios

NUTRITION (Per Day)
1,450 cal, 60 g pro, 138 g carb, 26 g fiber, 45 g sugars (3 g added sugars), 78.5 g fat (11.5 g sat fat), 1,320 mg sodium

WATER

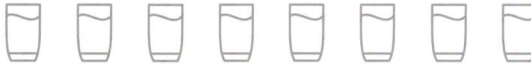

MOVEMENT/WORKOUT Y ☐ N ☐

ACTIVITY: _____

_____

_____

DURATION: _____

_____

_____

INTENSITY: _____

_____

SLEEP

Bedtime Last Night: _____ : _____

Wake Time This Morning: _____ : _____

_____

_____

_____

MOOD

_____

_____

_____

Day 5

BREAKFAST
Cocoa-Almond Smoothie (p. 65) + 1 piece avocado toast: Mash up ⅓ avocado, season with salt and pepper, and spread on top of 1 slice whole-grain bread.

LUNCH
Crispy Tofu Bowl (p. 81)

DINNER
Roasted Cauliflower Pizza (p. 89; 2 slices) + Greek Salad (p. 91)

SNACK
¼ cup hummus + ⅔ cup baby carrots

NUTRITION (Per Day) 1,665 cal, 62 g pro, 181 g carb, 50 g fiber, 50 g sugars (14 g added sugars), 81.5 g fat (15 g sat fat), 1,760 mg sodium

WATER

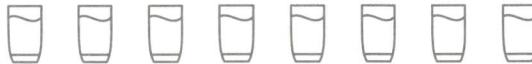

MOVEMENT/WORKOUT Y ☐ N ☐

ACTIVITY: _____

_____

_____

DURATION: _____

_____

_____

INTENSITY: _____

_____

SLEEP

Bedtime Last Night: _____ : _____

Wake Time This Morning: _____ : _____

_____

_____

_____

MOOD

😊 😐 ☹️

_____

_____

_____

_____

Day 6

BREAKFAST
Strawberry-Avocado Refresher (p. 64): Boost the nutrition of this delicious smoothie by adding 1 scoop of protein powder.

LUNCH
LEFTOVER Roasted Cauliflower Pizza (2 slices) + Greek Salad

DINNER
Charred Shrimp and Avocado Salad (p. 83)

SNACK
2 cups cubed melon + ½ oz pistachios

NUTRITION (Per Day)
1,445 cal, 62 g pro, 137 g carb, 28 g fiber, 62 g sugars (1 g added sugars), 79.5 g fat (14.5 g sat fat), 2,180 mg sodium

WATER

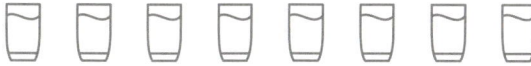

MOVEMENT/WORKOUT Y ☐ N ☐

ACTIVITY: _____

_____

_____

DURATION: _____

_____

_____

INTENSITY: _____

_____

_____

SLEEP

Bedtime Last Night: _____ : _____

Wake Time This Morning: _____ : _____

_____

_____

_____

MOOD

☺ ☹ ☹

_____

_____

_____

Day 7

BREAKFAST
Cocoa-Almond
Smoothie (p. 65)

LUNCH
Chickpea Pasta Salad
in a Jar (p. 79)

DINNER
LEFTOVER
Charred Shrimp and
Avocado Salad

SNACK
1 oz almonds
(about 23 pieces) +
1 medium banana

NUTRITION (Per Day)
1,535 cal, 50 g pro,
165 g carb, 51 g fiber,
54 g sugars (0 g added
sugars), 82 g fat (12 g sat
fat), 1,965 mg sodium

WATER

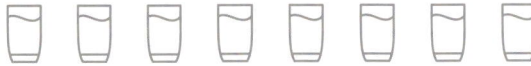

MOVEMENT/WORKOUT Y ☐ N ☐

ACTIVITY: _____

_____

_____

DURATION: _____

_____

_____

INTENSITY: _____

_____

_____

SLEEP

Bedtime Last Night: _____ : _____

Wake Time This Morning: _____ : _____

_____

_____

_____

MOOD

☺ ☻ ☹

_____

_____

_____

Week 2

Shopping List

→ **Before Your Grocery Run**

Check for leftovers from Week 1 before buying new ingredients from this shopping list.

PRODUCE

- 3 apples
- 2 avocados
- 6 medium bananas
- 1 pint blueberries
- 2 pieces butter lettuce
- 1 small bunch cilantro
- 2 limes
- 4 cloves garlic
- 1 small container grape tomatoes
- 2 cups grapes (about 1 lb)
- 1 small container cherry tomatoes
- 2 jalapeños
- 2 kiwis
- 1 large poblano pepper
- 2 red bell peppers
- 5 large scallions
- 1 large yellow onion
- 1 small red onion
- 1 8-oz bag raw sugar snap peas
- 1 16-oz bag spinach
- 4 tomatillos

DAIRY & REFRIGERATED

- 1 5.3-oz container plain Greek yogurt
- 1 5.3-oz container fat-free Greek yogurt
- 1 17.6-oz container 2% Greek yogurt
- 1 5.3-oz container vanilla Greek whole milk yogurt
- 1 10-oz bag frozen blueberries
- 1 10-oz bag frozen corn kernels
- 1 10-oz bag frozen mango chunks
- 1 oz sharp Cheddar
- 2 oz Gruyère cheese
- ½ dozen eggs
- 1 lb pizza dough
- 1 13.5-oz can unsweetened coconut milk, refrigerated
- 1 32-oz container unsweetened hemp milk
- 1 32-oz container unsweetened almond milk
- 1 12-oz container coconut water

MEATS & PROTEINS

- 1 3-oz pouch tuna fish
- 1 lb lean ground turkey
- 2 oz deli ham

PANTRY

- 1 8-inch whole-grain tortilla
- 2 oz (about 48 pieces) almonds
- 1 15-oz can canned pumpkin puree
- 4 oz raw cashews
- 1 small package quinoa
- 1 small bottle Dijon mustard
- 1 14.5-oz can fire-roasted diced tomatoes
- 1 small package flour
- 2 15-oz cans low-sodium black beans
- 1 8-oz container low-sodium chicken broth
- 1 small jar olive oil mayonnaise
- 1 small pouch pepitas
- 2 packets plain instant oatmeal
- 1 small jar pumpkin pie spice
- 3 slices sourdough
- 1 small pouch walnuts
- 3 slices whole-grain bread

Meal Plan

Day 8

BREAKFAST
PB + Banana-Berry Oatmeal (p. 35)

LUNCH
Lean, Mean, and Green Smoothie (p. 66) + 1 piece avocado toast (p. 35)

DINNER
Fiery Black Bean Soup (p. 93; 1 serving) + 1 slice sourdough

SNACK
23 almonds + 1 medium banana

Day 9

BREAKFAST
Blueberry Cashew Bliss (p. 67) + 1 hard-boiled egg

LUNCH
Tuna and Cheddar Wrap (p. 93) + 1 cup raw sugar snap peas

DINNER
Loaded Taco Bowl (p. 97; 1 serving)

SNACK
1 apple + 12 almonds

Day 10

BREAKFAST
Powerhouse Pumpkin Smoothie (p. 68)

LUNCH
LEFTOVER Loaded Taco Bowl (1 serving)

DINNER
LEFTOVER Fiery Black Bean Soup (1 serving) + 1 slice sourdough

SNACK
1 cup grapes + 1 oz cashews (about 20 whole pieces)

Day 11

BREAKFAST
Lean, Mean, and Green Smoothie (p. 66) + 1 piece avocado toast (p. 38)

LUNCH
LEFTOVER Fiery Black Bean Soup (1 serving) + 1 slice sourdough

DINNER
Sunny-Side-Up Pizza (p. 99; 1 serving)

SNACK
1 apple + 12 almonds

Day 12

BREAKFAST
Powerhouse Pumpkin Smoothie (p. 68)

LUNCH
Loaded Taco Bowl (p. 97; 1 serving)

DINNER
LEFTOVER Sunny-Side-Up Pizza (1 serving)

SNACK
1 cup grapes + 1 oz cashews (about 20 whole pieces)

Day 13

BREAKFAST
Blueberry Cashew Bliss Smoothie (p. 67) + 1 hard-boiled egg

LUNCH
LEFTOVER Sunny-Side-Up Pizza (1 serving)

DINNER
LEFTOVER Fiery Black Bean Soup (1 serving) + 1 slice sourdough

SNACK
1 apple + 1 oz cashews (about 20 whole pieces)

Day 14

BREAKFAST
PB + Banana-Berry Oatmeal (p. 41)

LUNCH
Turmeric Twist Smoothie (p. 70): Boost the nutrition of this delicious smoothie by adding 1 scoop protein powder.

DINNER
LEFTOVER Sunny-Side-Up Pizza (1 serving)

SNACK
1 5.3-oz vanilla Greek whole milk yogurt + 7 walnuts

Day 8

BREAKFAST
PB + Banana-Berry Oatmeal: In a small bowl, prepare 1 packet plain instant oatmeal according to package directions. Stir in 1 Tbsp creamy peanut butter, and add 1 banana (cut into bite-size pieces), and ½ cup blueberries.

LUNCH
Lean, Mean, and Green Smoothie (p. 66) + 1 piece avocado toast: Mash up ⅓ avocado, season with salt and pepper, and spread on top of 1 slice whole-grain bread.

DINNER
Fiery Black Bean Soup (p. 93; 1 serving) + 1 slice sourdough

SNACK
23 almonds + 1 medium banana

NUTRITION (Per Day) 1,620 cal, 82 g pro, 245 g carb, 49 g fiber, 81 g sugars (3 g added sugars), 46 g fat (6.5 g sat fat), 1,685 mg sodium

WATER

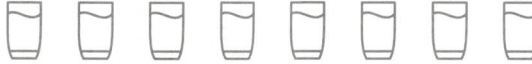

MOVEMENT/WORKOUT Y ☐ N ☐
ACTIVITY: _____
_____
_____

DURATION: _____
_____
_____

INTENSITY: _____
_____
_____

SLEEP
Bedtime Last Night: _____ : _____

Wake Time This Morning: _____ : _____
_____
_____
_____

MOOD
_____
_____
_____

Day 9

BREAKFAST
Blueberry Cashew
Bliss (p. 67) +
1 hard-boiled egg

LUNCH
Tuna and Cheddar
Wrap (p. 93) + 1 cup raw
sugar snap peas

DINNER
Loaded Taco Bowl
(p. 97; 1 serving)

SNACK
1 apple + 12 almonds

NUTRITION (Per Day)
1,480 cal, 87 g pro,
127 g carb, 22 g fiber,
42 g sugars (0 g added
sugars), 75 g fat
(17.5 g sat fat),
1,680 mg sodium

WATER

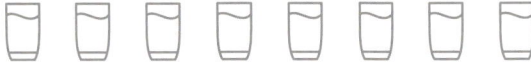

MOVEMENT/WORKOUT Y ☐ N ☐

ACTIVITY: _____
_____
_____

DURATION: _____
_____

INTENSITY: _____
_____

SLEEP

Bedtime Last Night: _____ : _____

Wake Time This Morning: _____ : _____

_____
_____
_____

MOOD

☺ ☺ ☹

_____
_____
_____

Day 10

BREAKFAST
Powerhouse Pumpkin
Smoothie (p. 68)

LUNCH
LEFTOVER Loaded Taco
Bowl (1 serving)

DINNER
LEFTOVER Fiery Black
Bean Soup (1 serving) +
1 slice sourdough

SNACK
1 cup grapes + 1 oz
cashews (about 20
whole pieces)

NUTRITION (Per Day)
1,585 cal, 85 g pro,
197 g carb, 37 g fiber,
67 g sugars (12 g added
sugars), 59 g fat (12 g sat
fat), 1,685 mg sodium

WATER

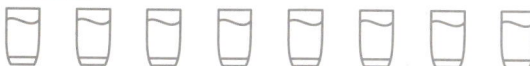

MOVEMENT/WORKOUT Y ☐ N ☐

ACTIVITY: _____

_____

_____

DURATION: _____

_____

_____

INTENSITY: _____

_____

_____

SLEEP

Bedtime Last Night: _____ : _____

Wake Time This Morning: _____ : _____

_____

_____

_____

_____

MOOD

☺ ☹ ☹

_____

_____

_____

_____

Day 11

BREAKFAST
Lean, Mean, and Green
Smoothie (p. 66) +
1 piece avocado toast:
Mash up ⅓ avocado,
season with salt and
pepper, and spread on
top of 1 slice whole-
grain bread.

LUNCH
LEFTOVER Fiery Black
Bean Soup (1 serving) +
1 slice sourdough

DINNER
Sunny-Side-Up Pizza
(p. 99; 1 serving)

SNACK
1 apple + 12 almonds

NUTRITION (Per Day)
1,645 cal, 91 g pro,
234 g carb, 41 g fiber,
64 g sugars (5 g added
sugars), 44 g fat
(10.5 g sat fat),
2,305 mg sodium

WATER

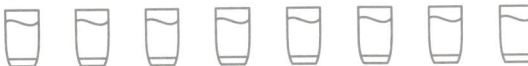

MOVEMENT/WORKOUT Y ☐ N ☐
ACTIVITY: _____

_____

_____

DURATION: _____

_____

_____

INTENSITY: _____

_____

SLEEP

Bedtime Last Night: _____ : _____

Wake Time This Morning: _____ : _____

_____

_____

_____

MOOD

☺ ☺ ☹

_____

_____

_____

_____

Day 12

BREAKFAST
Powerhouse Pumpkin
Smoothie (p. 68)

LUNCH
Loaded Taco Bowl
(p. 97; 1 serving)

DINNER
LEFTOVER Sunny-
Side-Up Pizza (1 serving)

SNACK
1 cup grapes + 1 oz
cashews (about 20
whole pieces)

NUTRITION (Per Day)
1,580 cal, 82 g pro,
174 g carb, 20 g fiber,
60 g sugars (14 g added
sugars), 67 g fat
(17 g sat fat),
1,445 mg sodium

WATER

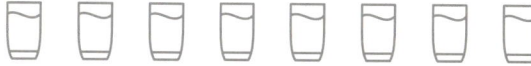

MOVEMENT/WORKOUT Y ☐ N ☐

ACTIVITY: _____

_____

DURATION: _____

_____

INTENSITY: _____

_____

SLEEP

Bedtime Last Night: _____ : _____

Wake Time This Morning: _____ : _____

_____

_____

_____

MOOD

☺ 😐 ☹

_____

_____

_____

Day 13

BREAKFAST
Blueberry Cashew Bliss
Smoothie (p. 67) +
1 hard-boiled egg

LUNCH
LEFTOVER Sunny-
Side-Up Pizza (1 serving)

DINNER
LEFTOVER Fiery Black
Bean Soup (1 serving) +
1 slice sourdough

SNACK
1 apple + 1 oz cashews
(about 20 whole pieces)

NUTRITION (Per Day)
1,505 cal, 69 g pro,
192 g carb, 31 g fiber,
46 g sugars (2 g added
sugars), 55.5 g fat
(15 g sat fat),
1,870 mg sodium

WATER

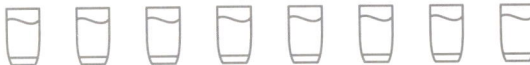

MOVEMENT/WORKOUT Y ☐ N ☐

ACTIVITY: _____

DURATION: _____

INTENSITY: _____

SLEEP

Bedtime Last Night: _____ : _____

Wake Time This Morning: _____ : _____

MOOD

Day 14

BREAKFAST
PB + Banana-Berry Oatmeal: In a small bowl, prepare 1 packet plain instant oatmeal according to package directions. Stir in 1 Tbsp creamy peanut butter, and add 1 banana (cut into bite-size pieces), and ½ cup blueberries. Pair it with 1 piece almond butter toast: Spread 1 Tbsp almond butter on 1 slice whole-grain bread.

LUNCH
Turmeric Twist Smoothie (p. 70): Boost the nutrition of this delicious smoothie by adding 1 scoop protein powder.

DINNER
LEFTOVER
Sunny-Side-Up Pizza (1 serving)

SNACK
1 5.3-oz vanilla Greek whole milk yogurt + 7 walnuts

NUTRITION (Per Day)
1,655 cal, 78 g pro, 203 g carb, 25 g fiber, 77 g sugars (13 g added sugars), 66 g fat (18.5 g sat fat), 1,260 mg sodium

WATER

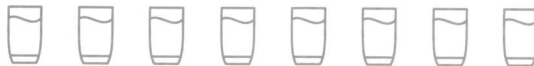

MOVEMENT/WORKOUT Y ☐ N ☐
ACTIVITY: _____

DURATION: _____

INTENSITY: _____

SLEEP

Bedtime Last Night: _____ : _____

Wake Time This Morning: _____ : _____

MOOD

Week 3

Shopping List

→ **Before Your Grocery Run**
Check for leftovers from Week 2 before buying new ingredients from this shopping list.

PRODUCE

2 apples

1 avocado

1 6-oz bag of baby spinach

3 bananas

2 Bartlett pears

1 head Boston lettuce

2 6-oz bags of butter lettuce

1 0.5-oz pack of mint leaves

1 medium-sized cantaloupe (about 3 lb)

1 bunch fresh cilantro leaves

1 lemon

2 limes

2 mangoes

1 1-in. piece ginger

1 clove garlic

2 plum tomatoes

1 pint grape tomatoes

1 naval orange

1 5-oz container mixed greens

1 small bunch parsley

2 Persian cucumbers

1 seedless cucumber

1 small bag shredded red cabbage

2 small red onions

1 small onion

1 small zucchini

DAIRY & REFRIGERATED

1 cheese stick

1 small container coconut water

½ dozen eggs

1 small package frozen mixed berries

1 small package frozen pineapple chunks

2 5.3-oz container vanilla Greek whole milk yogurt

1 30-oz container plain Greek yogurt

1 5.3-oz container plain low-fat yogurt

1 32-oz container unsweetened almond milk

1 10-oz bottle orange juice

MEATS & PROTEINS

2 14-oz blocks extra-firm tofu

8 oz roasted tempeh

12 oz large shrimp

PANTRY

1 15-oz can low-sodium chickpeas

1 small pouch raw cashews

1 small pouch roasted cashew halves

1 small pouch chopped toasted pecans

1 small pouch walnuts

1 small container cornstarch

1 small pouch dried cranberries

2 peanut butter squeeze packs

1 oz pistachios

1 small jar sliced pitted kalamata olives

1 32-oz container rolled oats

1 small container quick oats

1 small package quinoa

2 slices sourdough

1 small bottle Thai sweet chili sauce

2 slices whole-grain bread

4 whole-wheat pitas

Shredded, unsweetened coconut (optional)

Meal Plan

Day 15

BREAKFAST
Bingebuster
Smoothie (p. 69) +
1 hard-boiled egg

LUNCH
Crispy Tofu Bowl
(p. 81; 1 serving)

DINNER
Easy Tempeh Lettuce
Wraps (p. 101; 1 serving)
+ 1 oz cashews (about
20 whole pieces)

SNACK
2 cups cubed melon +
½ oz pistachios
(about 24 pieces)

Day 16

BREAKFAST
Pear-Spinach Smoothie
(p. 73) + 1 piece almond
butter toast (p. 45)

LUNCH
LEFTOVER
Easy Tempeh Lettuce
Wraps (1 serving)

DINNER
Shrimp, Avocado
and Egg Chopped Salad
(p. 103) + 1 slice
sourdough

SNACK
1 5.3-oz vanilla Greek
whole milk yogurt +
7 walnuts

Day 17

BREAKFAST
Bingebuster
Smoothie (p. 69) +
1 hard-boiled egg

LUNCH
Shrimp, Avocado
and Egg Chopped
Salad (p. 103) +
1 slice sourdough

DINNER
LEFTOVER
Crispy Tofu Bowl
(1 serving)

SNACK
2 cups cubed melon +
½ oz pistachios
(about 24 pieces)

Day 18

BREAKFAST
Pear-Spinach Smoothie
(p. 73)

LUNCH
Crispy Tofu Bowl
(p. 81; 1 serving)

DINNER
Greek Chickpea Tacos
(p. 105; 1 serving)

SNACK
1 cup fresh mango

Day 19

BREAKFAST
Four-Berry Belly Blast
(p. 71)

LUNCH
LEFTOVER
Greek Chickpea Tacos
(1 serving)

DINNER
Easy Tempeh Lettuce
Wraps (p. 101; 1 serving)

SNACK
1 banana + 1 peanut
butter squeeze pack

Day 20

BREAKFAST
Instant Oatmeal with
Cranberries and Pecans
(p. 107): Boost protein
of this hearty breakfast
by adding 1 Tbsp
almond butter.

LUNCH
Four-Berry Belly Blast
(p. 71) + 1 piece almond
butter toast (p. 49)

DINNER
LEFTOVER
Crispy Tofu Bowl
(1 serving)

SNACK
1 5.3-oz vanilla Greek
whole milk yogurt +
7 walnuts

Day 21

BREAKFAST
Banana Avocado Zinger
(p. 72): Boost nutrition
in this delicious
smoothie by adding
1 scoop protein powder.

LUNCH
Greek Chickpea Tacos
(p. 105; 1 serving)

DINNER
LEFTOVER
Easy Tempeh Lettuce
Wraps (1 serving) +
1 cup fresh mango

SNACK
1 banana + 1 peanut
butter squeeze pack

Day 15

BREAKFAST
Bingebuster
Smoothie (p. 69) +
1 hard-boiled egg

LUNCH
Crispy Tofu Bowl
(p. 81; 1 serving)

DINNER
Easy Tempeh Lettuce
Wraps (p. 101; 1 serving)
+ 1 oz cashews (about
20 whole pieces)

SNACK
2 cups cubed melon +
½ oz pistachios
(about 24 pieces)

NUTRITION (Per Day)
1,650 cal, 70 g pro,
185 g carb, 31 g fiber,
66 g sugars (10 g added
sugars), 76.5 g fat
(11.5 g sat fat),
880 mg sodium

WATER

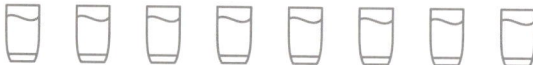

MOVEMENT/WORKOUT Y ☐ N ☐
ACTIVITY: _____

DURATION: _____

INTENSITY: _____

SLEEP
Bedtime Last Night: _____ : _____
Wake Time This Morning: _____ : _____

MOOD
☺ ☺ ☹

Day 16

BREAKFAST

Pear-Spinach Smoothie
(p. 73) + 1 piece almond
butter toast: Spread 1
Tbsp almond butter on 1
slice whole-grain bread.

LUNCH

LEFTOVER

Easy Tempeh Lettuce
Wraps (1 serving)

DINNER

Shrimp, Avocado,
and Egg Chopped Salad
(p. 103) + 1 slice
sourdough

SNACK

1 5.3-oz vanilla Greek
whole milk yogurt +
7 walnuts

NUTRITION (Per Day)
1,620 cal, 108 g pro,
160 g carb, 29 g fiber,
54 g sugars (11 g added
sugars), 69 g fat
(16 g sat fat),
1,600 mg sodium

WATER

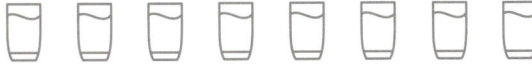

MOVEMENT/WORKOUT Y ☐ N ☐

ACTIVITY: _____

_____

_____

DURATION: _____

_____

_____

INTENSITY: _____

_____

_____

SLEEP

Bedtime Last Night: _____ : _____

Wake Time This Morning: _____ : _____

_____

_____

_____

MOOD

☺ ☺ ☹

_____

_____

_____

_____

Day 17

BREAKFAST
Bingebuster
Smoothie (p. 69) +
1 hard-boiled egg

LUNCH
Shrimp, Avocado,
and Egg Chopped
Salad (p. 103) +
1 slice sourdough

DINNER
LEFTOVER
Crispy Tofu Bowl
(1 serving)

SNACK
2 cups cubed melon +
½ oz pistachios
(about 24 pieces)

NUTRITION (Per Day)
1,675 cal, 92 g pro,
179 g carb, 29 g fiber,
67 g sugars (10 g added
sugars), 72.5 g fat
(11 g sat fat),
1,470 mg sodium

WATER

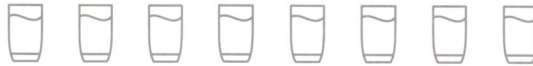

MOVEMENT/WORKOUT Y ☐ N ☐
ACTIVITY: _____
_____
_____

DURATION: _____
_____
_____

INTENSITY: _____
_____
_____

SLEEP
Bedtime Last Night: _____ : _____
Wake Time This Morning: _____ : _____
_____
_____
_____

MOOD
☺ ☺ ☹
_____
_____
_____

Day 18

BREAKFAST
Pear-Spinach Smoothie
(p. 73)

LUNCH
Crispy Tofu Bowl
(p. 81; 1 serving)

DINNER
Greek Chickpea Tacos
(p. 105; 1 serving)

SNACK
1 cup fresh mango

NUTRITION (Per Day)
1,355 cal, 64 g pro,
171 g carb, 24 g fiber,
68 g sugars (10 g added
sugars), 47.5 g fat
(10.5 g sat fat),
850 mg sodium

WATER

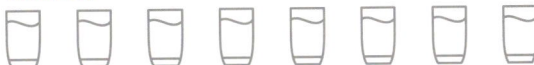

MOVEMENT/WORKOUT Y ☐ N ☐

ACTIVITY: _____
_____
_____

DURATION: _____
_____
_____

INTENSITY: _____
_____

SLEEP

Bedtime Last Night: _____ : _____

Wake Time This Morning: _____ : _____

_____
_____
_____

MOOD

☺ ☺ ☹

_____
_____
_____
_____

Day 19

BREAKFAST
Four-Berry Belly Blast
(p. 71)

LUNCH
LEFTOVER
Greek Chickpea Tacos
(1 serving)

DINNER
Easy Tempeh Lettuce
Wraps (p. 101; 1 serving)

SNACK
1 banana + 1 peanut
butter squeeze pack

NUTRITION (Per Day)
1,340 cal, 56 g pro,
175 g carb, 29 g fiber,
62 g sugars (0 g added
sugars), 50.5 g fat
(11.5 g sat fat),
1,175 mg sodium

WATER

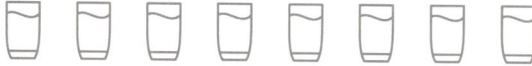

MOVEMENT/WORKOUT Y ☐ N ☐

ACTIVITY: _____

_____

_____

DURATION: _____

_____

_____

INTENSITY: _____

_____

_____

SLEEP

Bedtime Last Night: _____ : _____

Wake Time This Morning: _____ : _____

_____

_____

_____

MOOD

☺ ☻ ☹

_____

_____

_____

_____

Day 20

BREAKFAST
Instant Oatmeal with Cranberries and Pecans (p. 107): Boost protein of this hearty breakfast by adding 1 Tbsp almond butter.

LUNCH
Four-Berry Belly Blast (p. 71) + 1 piece almond butter toast: Spread 1 Tbsp almond butter on 1 slice whole-grain bread.

DINNER
LEFTOVER
Crispy Tofu Bowl (1 serving)

SNACK
1 5.3-oz vanilla Greek whole milk yogurt + 7 walnuts

NUTRITION (Per Day)
1,545 cal, 68 g pro, 178 g carb, 28 g fiber, 72 g sugars (27 g added sugars), 66.5 g fat (9.5 g sat fat), 585 mg sodium

WATER

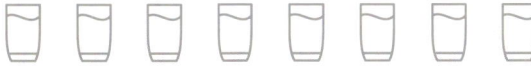

MOVEMENT/WORKOUT Y ☐ N ☐

ACTIVITY: _____

_____

_____

DURATION: _____

_____

_____

INTENSITY: _____

_____

_____

SLEEP

Bedtime Last Night: _____ : _____

Wake Time This Morning: _____ : _____

_____

_____

_____

MOOD

_____

_____

_____

Day 21

BREAKFAST
Banana Avocado Zinger (p. 72): Boost nutrition in this delicious smoothie by adding 1 scoop protein powder.

LUNCH
Greek Chickpea Tacos (p. 105; 1 serving)

DINNER
LEFTOVER
Easy Tempeh Lettuce Wraps (1 serving) + 1 cup fresh mango

SNACK
1 banana + 1 peanut butter squeeze pack

NUTRITION (Per Day)
1,575 cal, 68 g pro, 191 g carb, 36 g fiber, 66 g sugars (0 g added sugars), 67 g fat (13 g sat fat), 1,250 mg sodium

WATER

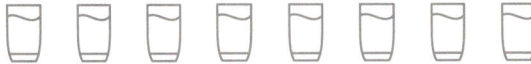

MOVEMENT/WORKOUT Y ☐ N ☐

ACTIVITY: _____

DURATION: _____

INTENSITY: _____

SLEEP

Bedtime Last Night: _____ : _____

Wake Time This Morning: _____ : _____

MOOD

Week 4

Shopping List

→ **Before Your Grocery Run**
Check for leftovers from Week 3 before buying new ingredients from this shopping list.

PRODUCE

- 1 5-oz bag arugula
- 2 avocados
- 1 small package baby carrots
- 4 bananas
- 1 12-oz bag cauliflower florets
- 1 pint grape tomatoes
- 1 tomato
- 1 small bulb fennel
- 1 fresh mango
- 3 cloves garlic
- 1 lb green or wax beans, or a combination
- 1½ bunches kale
- 4 kiwis
- 4 large sweet potatoes
- 2 lemons
- 12 oz mini sweet peppers
- 1 naval orange
- 4 small Persian cucumbers
- 1 small pink grapefruit
- 1 small red onion

DAIRY & REFRIGERATED

- 1 stick butter
- 1 cheese stick
- 1 small container coconut water
- 1 small container feta cheese
- ½ dozen eggs
- 1 quart fat-free milk
- 1 small package frozen blueberries
- 1 small package frozen raspberries
- 1 small package frozen strawberries
- 1 small package frozen mixed berries
- 1 5.3-oz container vanilla low-fat yogurt
- 1 16-oz container Greek whole milk yogurt
- 1 small container hummus
- 1 small package reduced-fat Cheddar cheese

MEATS & PROTEINS

- 2 5-oz skinless salmon fillets
- 2 6-oz boneless, skinless chicken breasts
- 1½ lb strip or sirloin steak

PANTRY

- 1 oz (or 20 pieces) almonds
- 1 15-oz can lentils
- 1 8-oz bottle pomegranate juice
- 1 small container quick-cooking farro
- 1 small jar fennel seeds
- 1 10-oz container golden raisins
- 1 15-oz can pinto beans
- 2 slices sourdough
- 1 5-oz container sunflower seeds
- 1 small container toasted pine nuts
- 1 small container toasted pistachios
- 1 small package walnuts
- 1 small bottle white wine vinegar
- 3 slices whole-grain bread
- 1 whole-wheat English muffin
- 1 small bottle Worcestershire sauce

Meal Plan

Day 22

BREAKFAST
Protein Power
Smoothie (p. 75)

LUNCH
Kale and Cauliflower
Roasted Salad (p. 109;
1 serving) + 1 piece
avocado toast (p. 53)

DINNER
Veggie Medley on
Sweet Potatoes (p. 111;
1 serving)

SNACK
1 banana + 10 almonds

Day 23

BREAKFAST
Strawberry-Chia
Smoothie (p. 74) +
1 hard-boiled egg

LUNCH
LEFTOVER
Veggie Medley on Sweet
Potatoes (1 serving)

DINNER
Salmon with Grapefruit
and Lentil Salad (p. 113)
+ 1 slice sourdough

SNACK
¼ cup hummus +
⅔ cup baby carrots

Day 24

BREAKFAST
Protein Power
Smoothie (p. 75)

LUNCH
Salmon with Grapefruit
and Lentil Salad (p. 113)
+ 1 slice sourdough

DINNER
LEFTOVER
Veggie Medley on Sweet
Potatoes (1 serving)

SNACK
½ cup Greek whole milk
yogurt + 7 walnuts

Day 25

BREAKFAST
Strawberry-Chia
Smoothie (p. 74)

LUNCH
LEFTOVER Kale and
Cauliflower Roasted
Salad (1 serving) +
1 piece avocado toast
(p. 56)

DINNER
Steak with Green
Beans, Fennel & Farro
(p. 115; 1 serving)

SNACK
1 banana + 10 almonds

Day 26

BREAKFAST
Banana-Almond Protein
Smoothie (p. 76) +
1 hard-boiled egg

LUNCH
LEFTOVER Steak with
Green Beans, Fennel &
Farro (1 serving)

DINNER
Greek Chicken Grain
Bowl (p. 116; 1 serving)

SNACK
½ cup Greek whole milk
yogurt + 7 walnuts

Day 27

BREAKFAST
Hearty Breakfast Egg
Sandwich (p. 117)

LUNCH
Banana-Almond Protein
Smoothie (p. 76) +
1 piece avocado toast
(p. 58)

DINNER
Steak with Green
Beans, Fennel & Farro
(p. 115; 1 serving)

SNACK
1 naval orange +
1 cheese stick

Day 28

BREAKFAST
Pomegranate-Berry
Smoothie (p. 77):
Boost nutrition of
this delicious smoothie
by adding 1 scoop
protein powder.

LUNCH
LEFTOVER
Greek Chicken Grain
Bowl (1 serving)

DINNER
LEFTOVER
Veggie Medley on Sweet
Potatoes (1 serving) +
1 cup fresh mango

SNACK
¼ cup hummus +
⅔ cup baby carrots

Day 22

BREAKFAST
Protein Power
Smoothie (p. 75)

LUNCH
Kale and Cauliflower
Roasted Salad (p. 109;
1 serving) + 1 piece
avocado toast: Mash up
⅓ avocado, season with
salt and pepper, and
spread on top of 1 slice
whole-grain bread.

DINNER
Veggie Medley on
Sweet Potatoes (p. 111;
1 serving)

SNACK
1 banana + 10 almonds

NUTRITION (Per Day)
1,605 cal, 67 g pro,
194 g carb, 36 g fiber,
75 g sugars (3 g added
sugars), 72 g fat
(13.5 g sat fat),
1,540 mg sodium

WATER

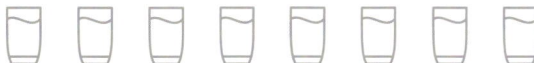

MOVEMENT/WORKOUT Y ☐ **N** ☐
ACTIVITY: _____
_____
_____

DURATION: _____
_____
_____

INTENSITY: _____
_____

SLEEP

Bedtime Last Night: _____ : _____
Wake Time This Morning: _____ : _____

MOOD

Day 23

BREAKFAST
Strawberry-Chia
Smoothie (p. 74) +
1 hard-boiled egg

LUNCH
LEFTOVER
Veggie Medley
on Sweet Potatoes
(1 serving)

DINNER
Salmon with Grapefruit
and Lentil Salad (p. 113)
+ 1 slice sourdough

SNACK
¼ cup hummus +
⅔ cup baby carrots

NUTRITION (Per Day)
1,500 cal, 80 g pro,
177 g carb, 33 g fiber,
60 g sugars (0 g added
sugars), 56 g fat
(15 g sat fat),
1,785 mg sodium

WATER

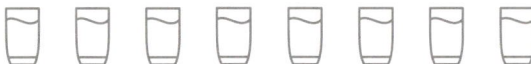

MOVEMENT/WORKOUT Y ☐ N ☐

ACTIVITY: _____

_____

_____

DURATION: _____

_____

_____

INTENSITY: _____

_____

_____

SLEEP

Bedtime Last Night: _____ : _____

Wake Time This Morning: _____ : _____

_____

_____

_____

_____

MOOD

☺ ☻ ☹

_____

_____

_____

_____

Day 24

BREAKFAST
Protein Power
Smoothie (p. 75)

LUNCH
Salmon with Grapefruit
and Lentil Salad (p. 113)
+ 1 slice sourdough

DINNER
LEFTOVER
Veggie Medley on Sweet
Potatoes (1 serving)

SNACK
½ cup Greek whole milk
yogurt + 7 walnuts

NUTRITION (Per Day)
1,525 cal, 100 g pro,
165 g carb, 27 g fiber,
60 g sugars (0 g added
sugars), 56 g fat
(12.5 g sat fat),
1,500 mg sodium

WATER

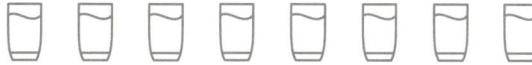

MOVEMENT/WORKOUT Y ☐ N ☐

ACTIVITY: _____

_____

_____

DURATION: _____

_____

INTENSITY: _____

_____

SLEEP

Bedtime Last Night: _____ : _____

Wake Time This Morning: _____ : _____

_____

_____

_____

MOOD

😊 😐 ☹

_____

_____

_____

_____

Day 25

BREAKFAST
Strawberry-Chia
Smoothie (p. 74)

LUNCH
LEFTOVER Kale and
Cauliflower Roasted
Salad (1 serving) +
1 piece avocado toast:
Mash up ⅓ avocado,
season with salt and
pepper, and spread on
top of 1 slice whole-
grain bread.

DINNER
Steak with Green
Beans, Fennel & Farro
(p. 115; 1 serving)

SNACK
1 banana + 10 almonds

NUTRITION (Per Day)
1,615 cal, 69 g pro,
164 g carb, 38 g fiber,
68 g sugars (4 g added
sugars), 85.5 g fat
(17.5 g sat fat),
1,305 mg sodium

WATER

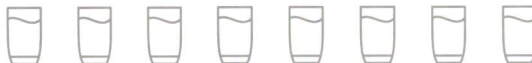

MOVEMENT/WORKOUT Y ☐ N ☐

ACTIVITY: _____

_____

DURATION: _____

_____

INTENSITY: _____

_____

SLEEP

Bedtime Last Night: _____ : _____

Wake Time This Morning: _____ : _____

MOOD

Day 26

BREAKFAST
Banana-Almond Protein Smoothie (p. 76) + 1 hard-boiled egg

LUNCH
LEFTOVER Steak with Green Beans, Fennel & Farro (1 serving)

DINNER
Greek Chicken Grain Bowl (p. 116; 1 serving)

SNACK
½ cup Greek whole milk yogurt + 7 walnuts

NUTRITION (Per Day)
1,645 cal, 119 g pro, 101 g carb, 19 g fiber, 31 g sugars (1 g added sugars), 87.5 g fat (17.5 g sat fat), 1,230 mg sodium

WATER

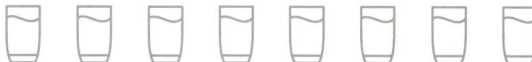

MOVEMENT/WORKOUT Y ☐ N ☐

ACTIVITY: _____

_____

DURATION: _____

_____

INTENSITY: _____

_____

SLEEP

Bedtime Last Night: _____ : _____

Wake Time This Morning: _____ : _____

MOOD

Day 27

BREAKFAST
Hearty Breakfast Egg Sandwich (p. 117)

LUNCH
Banana-Almond Protein Smoothie (p. 76) +
1 piece avocado toast: Mash up ⅓ avocado, season with salt and pepper, and spread on top of 1 slice whole-grain bread.

DINNER
Steak with Green Beans, Fennel & Farro (p. 115; 1 serving)

SNACK
1 naval orange +
1 cheese stick

NUTRITION (Per Day)
1,590 cal, 99 g pro,
134 g carb, 30 g fiber,
46 g sugars (9 g added sugars), 79.5 g fat
(21 g sat fat),
2,060 mg sodium

WATER

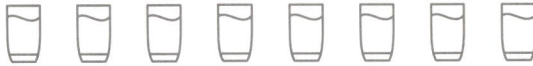

MOVEMENT/WORKOUT Y ☐ N ☐

ACTIVITY: _____

_____

_____

DURATION: _____

_____

INTENSITY: _____

_____

SLEEP

Bedtime Last Night: _____ : _____

Wake Time This Morning: _____ : _____

MOOD

☺ ☺ ☹

Day 28

BREAKFAST
Pomegranate-Berry
Smoothie (p. 77):
Boost nutrition of
this delicious smoothie
by adding 1 scoop
protein powder.

LUNCH
LEFTOVER
Greek Chicken Grain
Bowl (1 serving)

DINNER
LEFTOVER
Veggie Medley
on Sweet Potatoes
(1 serving) +
1 cup fresh mango

SNACK
¼ cup hummus +
⅔ cup baby carrots

NUTRITION (Per Day)
1,630 cal, 89 g pro,
201 g carb, 29 g fiber,
91 g sugars (8 g added
sugars), 55.5 g fat
(11.5 g sat fat),
1,710 mg sodium

WATER

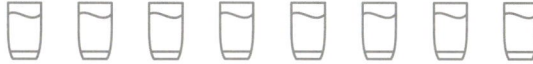

MOVEMENT/WORKOUT Y ☐ N ☐
ACTIVITY: _____
_____
_____

DURATION: _____
_____
_____

INTENSITY: _____
_____
_____

SLEEP
Bedtime Last Night: _____ : _____
Wake Time This Morning: _____ : _____
_____
_____
_____
_____

MOOD

_____
_____
_____
_____

CHAPTER 4

Meal Plan Recipes

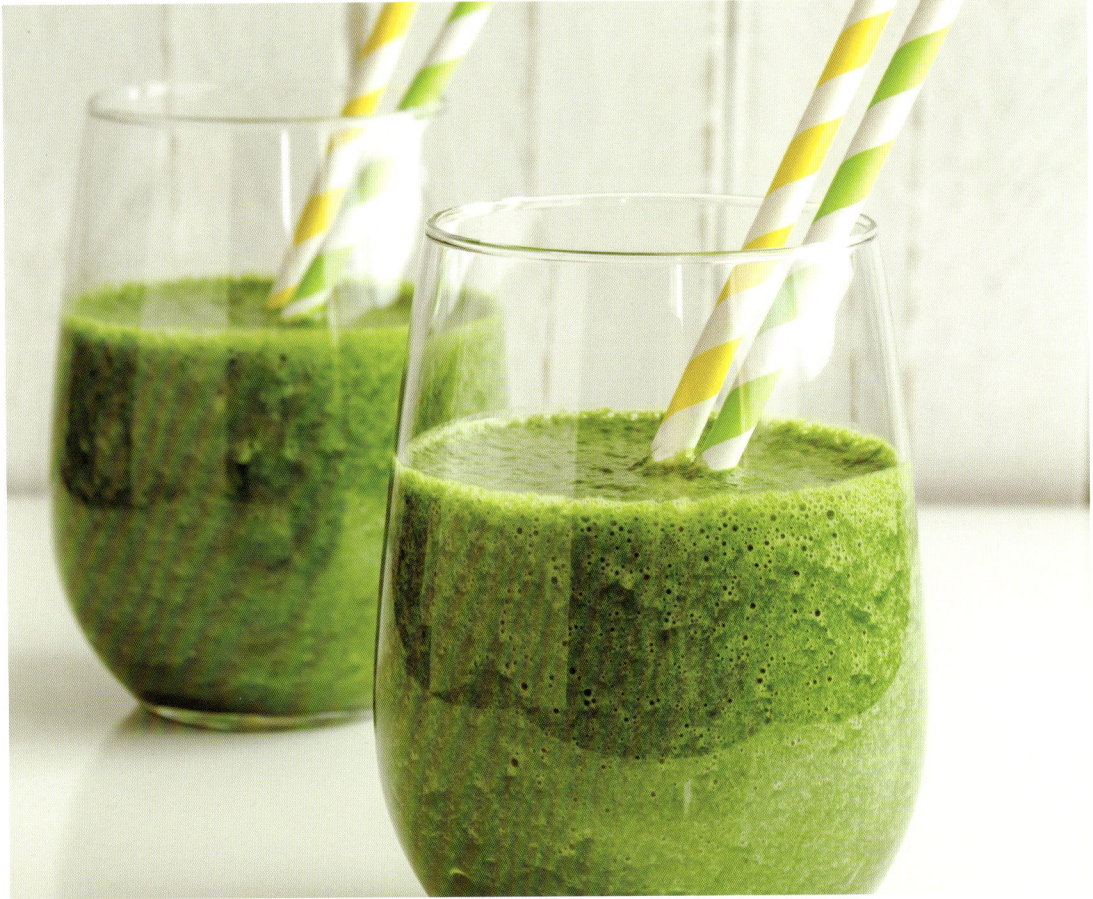

Creamy Kale Smoothie

HIGH FIBER

TOTAL **5 MIN**. // SERVES **1**

Packed with protein and probiotics, Greek yogurt is a natural in healthy-gut smoothies. And pineapple contains bromelain, an enzyme that helps break down protein and may help reduce bloating. Together, they make this one a sweet way to be good to your gut.

½ **cup plain Greek yogurt**
½ **cup unsweetened almond milk**
1 **tsp honey**
1 **cup kale, coarsely chopped**
1½ **cups frozen
    pineapple chunks**

In a blender, combine all ingredients and puree until smooth.

PER SERVING
295 cal, 14 g pro,
45 g carb, 5 g fiber,
36 g sugars
(6 g added sugars),
8.5 g fat
(3 g sat fat),
145 mg sodium

Sweet 'n' Spicy Tropical Smoothie

TOTAL **10 MIN.** // SERVES **1**

Combining the electrolytes in coconut water, the spicy kick from cayenne, and the muscle-repairing benefits of whey protein, this post-workout smoothie will help your muscles recover.

- 2 **Tbsp coconut water**
- ½ **Tbsp lemon juice**
- **Pinch cayenne powder**
- ½- **in. piece fresh ginger, peeled and chopped**
- ⅛ **ripe avocado, pitted and peeled**
- 1 **Tbsp unsweetened whey protein powder**
- ¼ **cup frozen pineapple or mango chunks**

In a blender, combine all ingredients and puree until smooth.

PER SERVING 95 cal, 5 g pro, 11 g carb, 2 g fiber, 3 g sugars (0 g added sugars), 4 g fat (0.5 g sat fat), 15 mg sodium

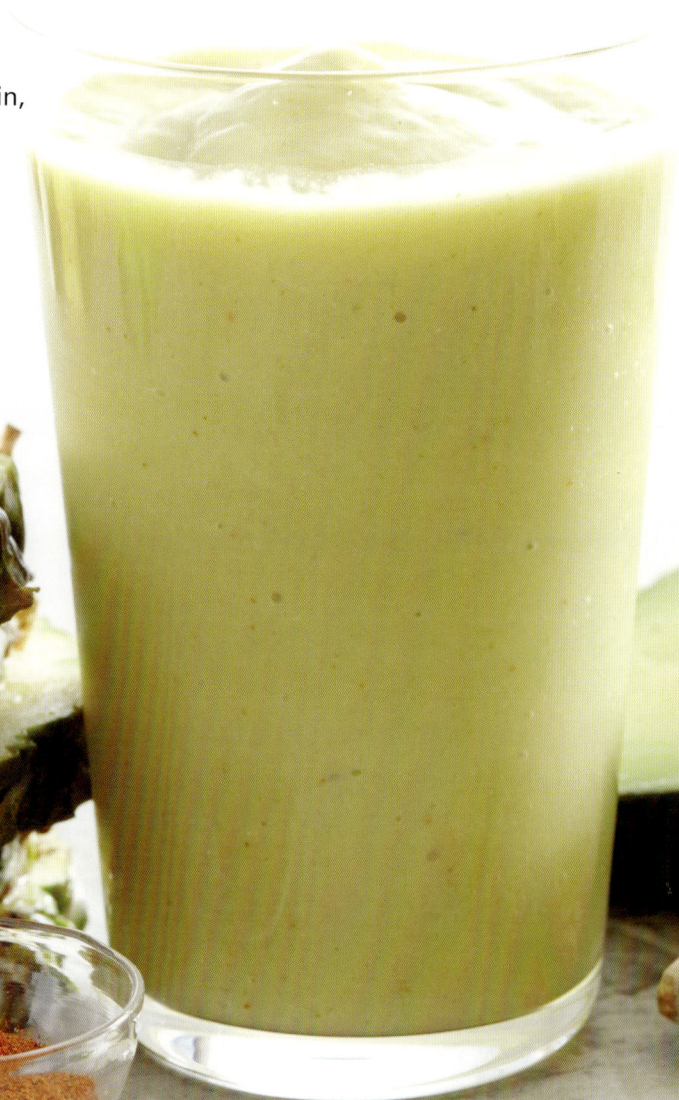

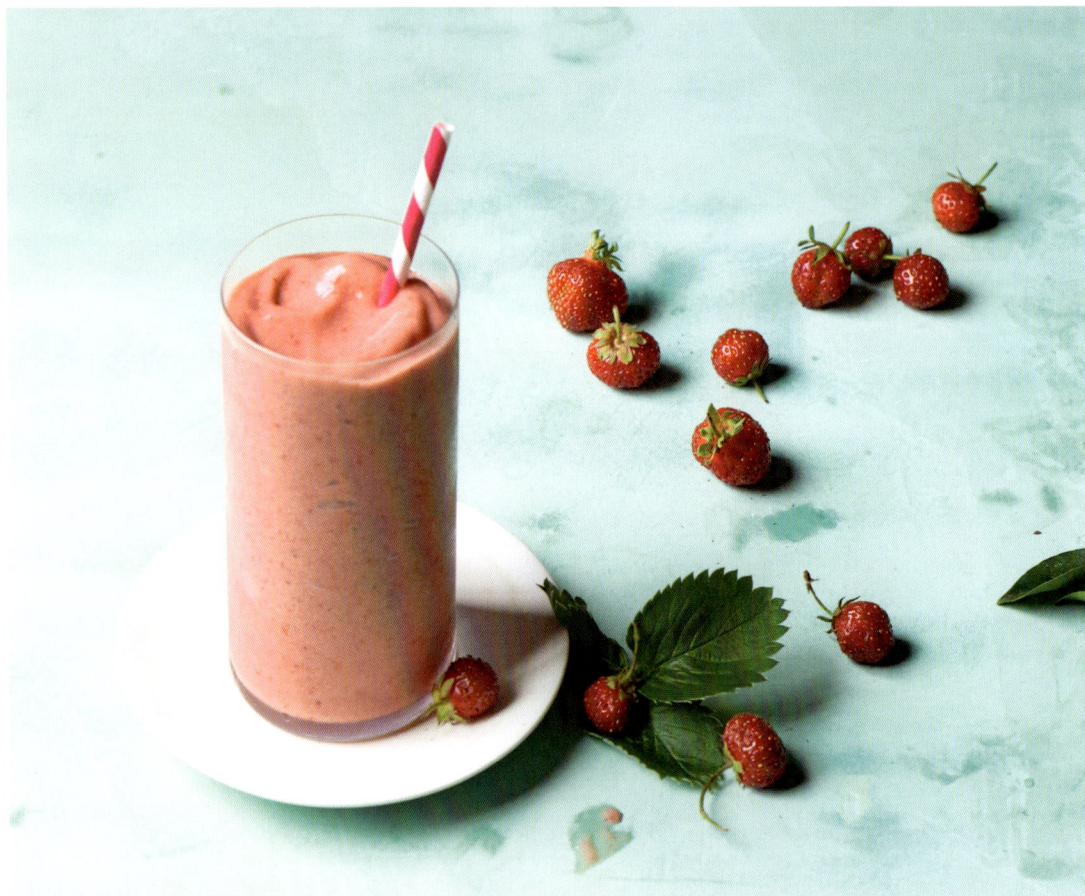

Strawberry-Avocado Refresher

VEGAN
HIGH FIBER

TOTAL **5 MIN**. // SERVES **1**

Pairing strawberries and avocados makes this creamy and delicious smoothie a great source of potassium—a nutrient that counteracts bloat-inducing sodium in your diet— which can help you lose water weight.

Juice of half a lime
1 **cup halved strawberries**
½ **avocado, pitted and peeled**
½ **large frozen banana**
Handful of ice

In a blender, combine all ingredients and puree until smooth.

PER SERVING
275 cal, 4 g pro,
38 g carb, 12 g
fiber, 17 g sugars
(0 g added sugars),
15.5 g fat (2 g sat
fat), 10 mg sodium

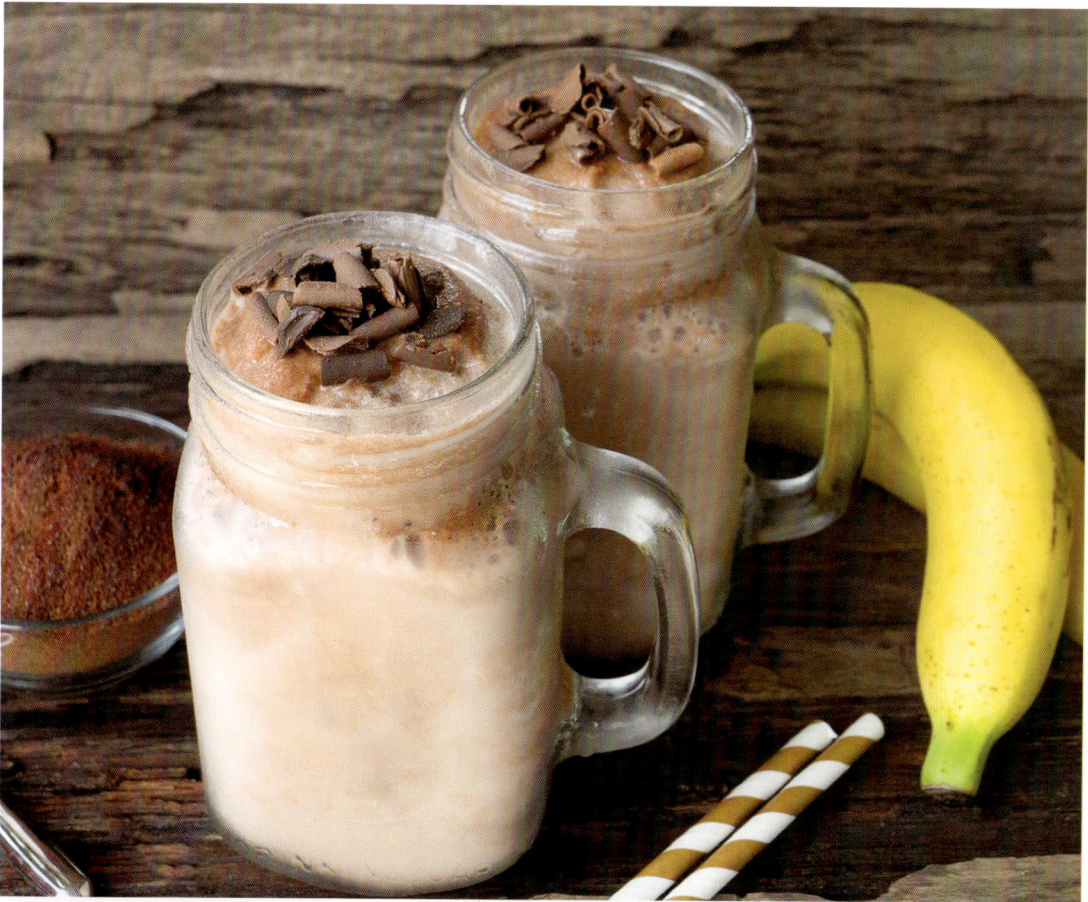

Cocoa-Almond Smoothie

HIGH FIBER

TOTAL **5 MIN**. // SERVES **1**

Nuts, in general, are good for your gut—and almonds are the fiber champs. Pair them with cocoa, which clocks in at almost 2 grams of fiber per tablespoon, and you have yourself a rich and filling smoothie that may help you eat less and stay satisfied longer.

½ **cup unsweetened almond milk**
1 **Tbsp unsweetened cocoa powder**
1 **Tbsp almond butter**
1½ **pitted dates**
1 **ripe banana (preferably frozen), sliced into 1-in. rounds (see p. 8 for tips on freezing bananas)**
½ **cup ice cubes**
Dark chocolate shavings, optional

In a blender, combine all ingredients and puree until smooth. Pour into a glass or jar, add chocolate shavings on top, if using, and serve.

PER SERVING
260 cal, 6 g pro,
42 g carb, 28 g
fiber, 22 g sugars
(0 g added sugars),
11 g fat (1 g sat fat),
70 mg sodium

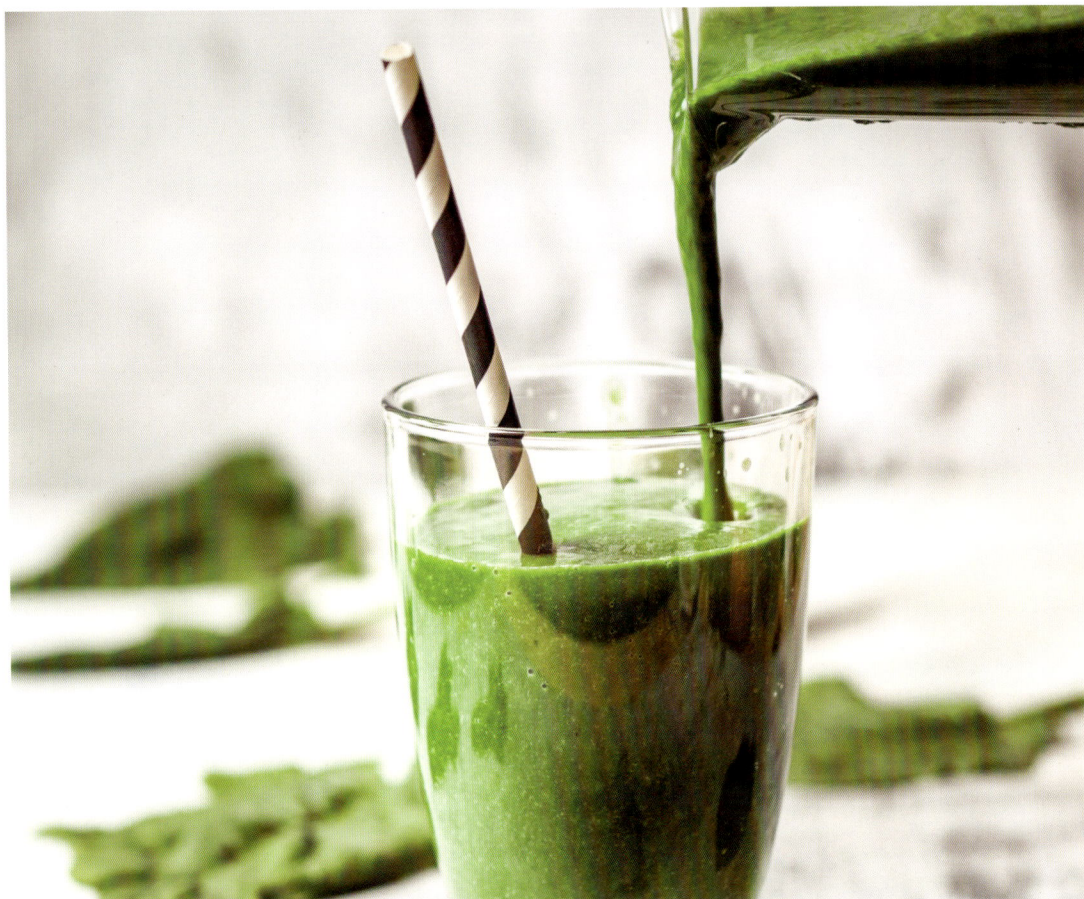

Lean, Mean & Green Machine

VEGAN
PROTEIN-PACKED
HIGH FIBER

TOTAL **5 MIN**. // SERVES **1**

If you're looking for a post-workout recovery drink, this smoothie is it. Carbohydrates (in the fruit and coconut water) help replenish the energy you burn and protein powder helps with muscle recovery.

½ cup coconut water
1 cup unsweetened almond milk
1 banana
1 kiwi, peeled and cut into pieces
1 cup spinach
1 scoop vanilla whey protein powder

In a blender, combine all ingredients and puree until smooth.

PER SERVING
345 cal, 34 g pro,
47 g carb, 7 g fiber,
27 g sugars
(0 g added sugars),
4 g fat (0.5 g
sat fat), 400 mg
sodium

HIGH FIBER

Blueberry Cashew Bliss

TOTAL **5 MIN**. // SERVES **1**

Blueberries make the list of superfoods because they're packed with antioxidants that help your overall health. Recent studies show that adults who ate blueberries had up to a 26% lower risk of type 2 diabetes than those who didn't. That's pretty impressive for a tiny berry that has only 80 calories per cup!

¼ **cup unsweetened hemp milk**
¼ **cup plain Greek yogurt**
½ **Tbsp hulled hemp seeds**
½ **tsp chia seeds**
2 **Tbsp raw cashews**
½ **cup frozen blueberries**
¼ **banana, sliced and frozen**
¼ **cup ice**

In a blender, combine all ingredients and puree until smooth.

PER SERVING 260 cal, 11 g pro, 25 g carb, 5 g fiber, 13 g sugars (0 g added sugars), 14.5 g fat (3 g sat fat), 55 mg sodium

HIGH FIBER· PROTEIN-PACKED

Powerhouse Pumpkin Smoothie

TOTAL **5 MIN**. // SERVES **1**

Pumpkin is rich in satiating fiber and low in calories, so it's a great option for weight-loss-friendly shakes. The pumpkin pie spice adds just enough warmth to give you all the fall feels.

7	oz 2% Greek yogurt
½	cup water
2	Tbsp ground flaxseed
1	Tbsp pure maple syrup
½	tsp pumpkin pie spice
½	cup canned pumpkin puree
¼	avocado, peeled

In a blender, combine all ingredients and puree until smooth.

PER SERVING 390 cal, 21 g pro, 40 g carb, 10 g fiber, 26 g sugars (12 g added sugars), 18 g fat (4 g sat fat), 80 mg sodium

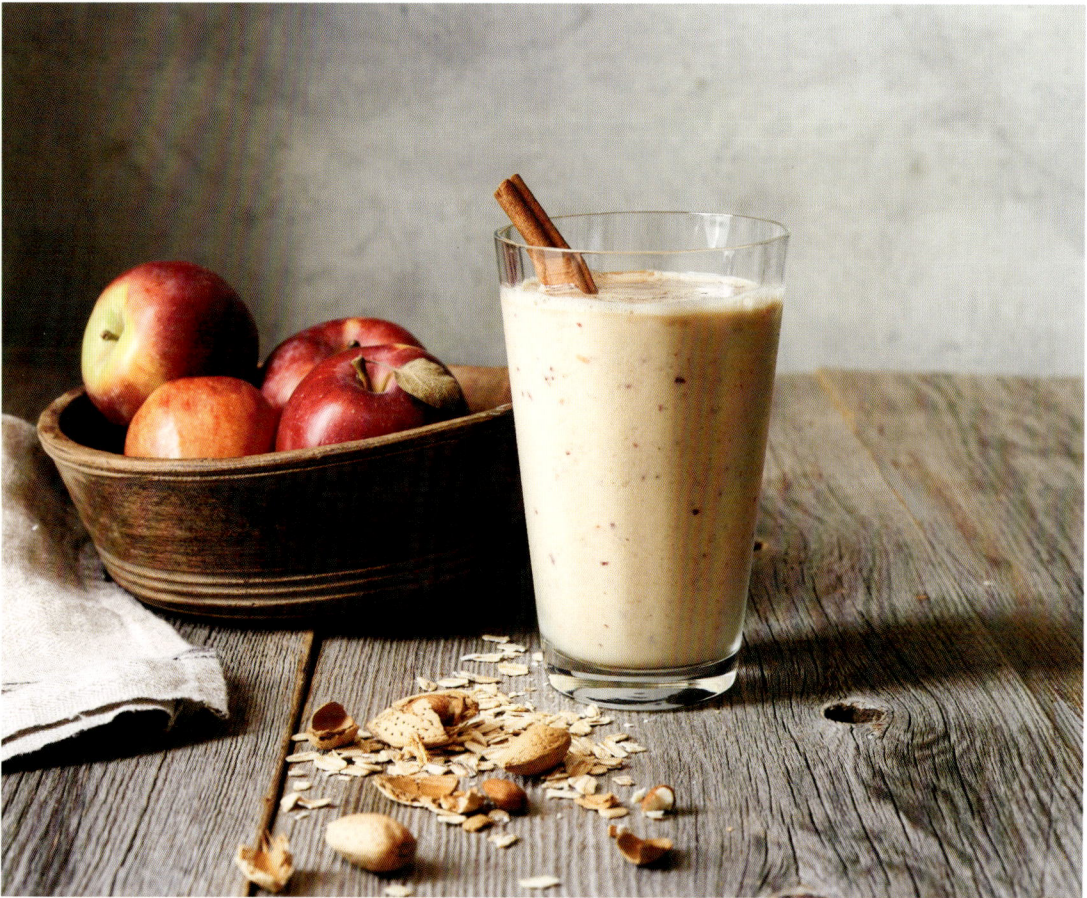

Bingebuster Smoothie

VEGAN
HIGH FIBER

TOTAL **5 MIN.** // SERVES **1**

When you have the urge to run straight to the nearest cupcake, turn to this fiber-packed smoothie. The apple and oats make you feel full, while the cinnamon and apple cider vinegar help stabilize blood sugar. The protein in the almond butter adds to the feeling of satiety, helping you forget all about that sugar craving.

¾ **cup unsweetened almond milk**

1 **tsp apple cider vinegar**

1 **Tbsp almond butter**

1 **tsp ground cinnamon**

¼ **cups rolled oats**

1 **apple, cored and chopped**

In a blender, combine all ingredients and puree until smooth.

PER SERVING
305 cal, 7 g pro, 45 g carb, 10 g fiber, 20 g sugars (0 g added sugars), 13 g fat (1 g sat fat), 140 mg sodium

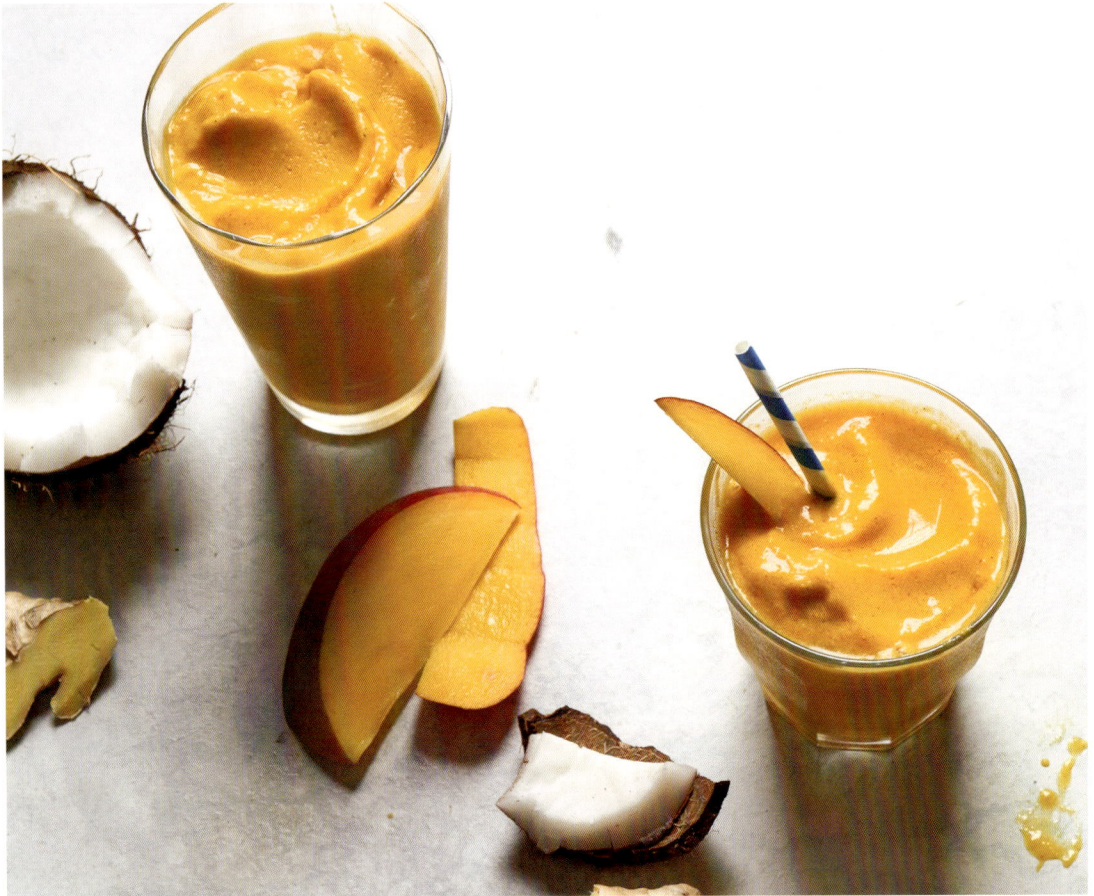

Turmeric Twist Smoothie

HIGH FIBER

TOTAL **5 MIN**. // SERVES **1**

Turmeric is a super spice that does it all—it can boost your memory, ease joint pain, ward off heart disease, and even turn bland dishes into nutritional gold. It also improves insulin resistance and increases metabolism which aids in weight loss.

½ **cup refrigerated unsweetened coconut milk**

¼ **cup water**

1 **Tbsp hemp seeds**

½ **tsp ground ginger**

½ **tsp ground turmeric**

1 **cup frozen mango chunks**

Handful of ice

Honey, to taste (optional)

In a blender, combine all ingredients and puree until smooth. If you like, add honey to taste.

PER SERVING
260 cal, 5 g pro,
41 g carb, 5 g fiber,
31 g sugars
(0 g added sugars),
10 g fat (5 g sat
fat), 40 mg sodium

HIGH FIBER

Four-Berry Belly Blast

TOTAL **5 MIN**. // SERVES **1**

Try this healthy smoothie as a smart substitute for a sugary dessert. This slimming sipper is chock-full of four different berries and the health benefits that come with them.

- ½ **cup frozen mixed berries (blueberries, raspberries, blackberries, strawberries)**
- ¼ **cup plain low-fat yogurt**
- ½ **cup orange juice**
- **Shredded, unsweetened coconut (optional), for topping**

In a blender, combine all ingredients and puree until smooth. Serve with shredded coconut if desired.

If using coconut, place the shredded coconut in a bowl. Use a pastry brush or a paper towel to coat the inner and outer rim of a glass with honey or agave syrup. Dip glass in coconut to coat then carefully fill with smoothie and serve.

PER SERVING 240 cal, 10 g pro, 47 g carb, 7 g fiber, 31 g sugars (0 g added sugars), 2 g fat (1 g sat fat), 90 mg sodium

VEGAN   HIGH FIBER

Banana Avocado Zinger

TOTAL **10 MIN**. // SERVES **1**

Need a pre-workout pick-me-up? Get revved naturally with B vitamins, which are plentiful in bananas, avocado, spinach, and parsley. Pineapple provides manganese, a mineral that's essential for energy production.

- ¼ **cup chilled coconut water**
- 1 **Tbsp fresh lime juice**
- ¼ **cup parsley, chopped**
- ½ **small avocado, pitted and peeled**
- ¼ **cup baby spinach leaves**
- ½ **frozen banana, chopped**
- ¼ **cup frozen pineapple chunks**

In a blender, combine all ingredients and puree until smooth.

PER SERVING 215 cal, 3 g pro, 31 g carb, 8 g fiber, 11 g sugars (0 g added sugars), 11 g fat (2 g sat fat), 35 mg sodium

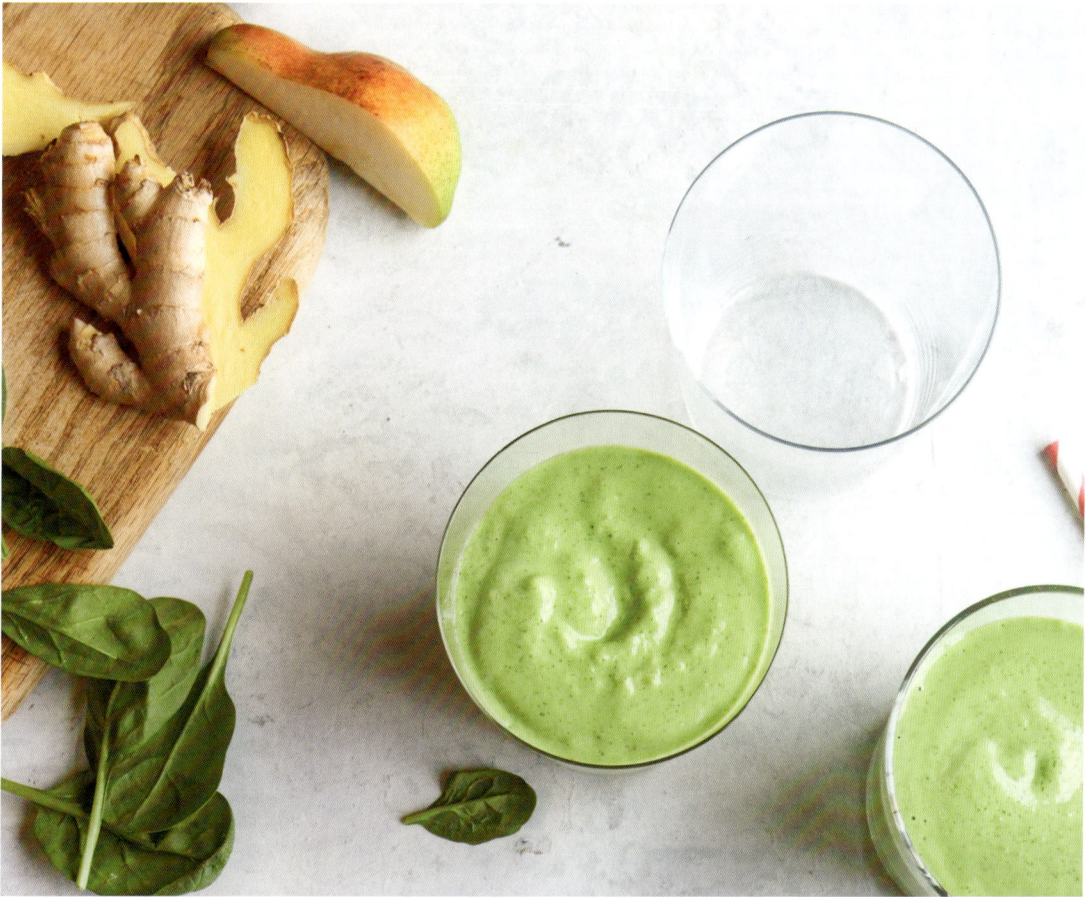

Pear-Spinach Smoothie

HIGH FIBER
PROTEIN-PACKED

TOTAL **10 MIN**. // SERVES **1**

Need to get things moving? Probiotic-rich yogurt can help keep you regular. And one medium pear boasts nearly 6 grams of fiber, making it a go-to ingredient when you need to go.

- ¾   **cup Greek yogurt**
- ½- **in. piece fresh ginger, peeled and grated**
- 1   **cup spinach**
- 1   **Bartlett pear, quartered and cored**
     Handful of ice

In a blender, combine all ingredients and puree until smooth.

PER SERVING
305 cal, 19 g pro, 36 g carb, 6 g fiber, 25 g sugars (0 g added sugars), 10 g fat (4.5 g sat fat), 90 mg sodium

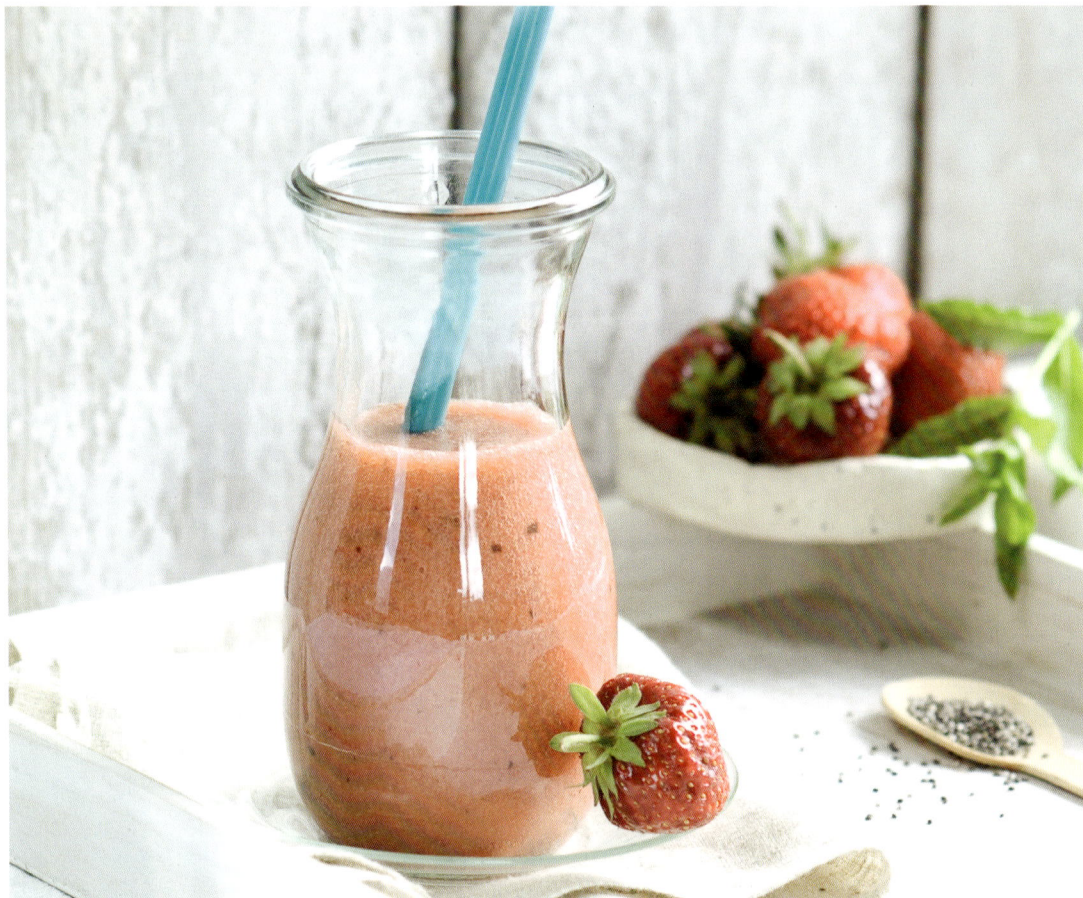

Strawberry-Chia Smoothie

HIGH FIBER

TOTAL **10 MIN**. // SERVES **1**

OJ isn't the only way to get your vitamin C in the morning. Kiwis and strawberries are also good sources, and this fruity blend with chia seeds is custom-made to rev up your day. The chia seeds hold on to water, making this an especially hydrating post-workout drink.

- ¾ **cup milk of your choice**
- 1 **Tbsp chia seeds**
- 1 **tsp ground ginger**
- 2 **kiwis, peeled and chopped**
- 1 **cup frozen strawberries**
- 4 **ice cubes**

In a blender, combine all ingredients and puree until smooth.

PER SERVING
305 cal, 10 g pro, 48 g carb, 11 g fiber, 28 g sugars (0 g added sugars), 10 g fat (4 g sat fat), 90 mg sodium

HIGH FIBER PROTEIN-PACKED

Protein Power Smoothie

TOTAL **5 MIN.** // SERVES **1**

Blend up this delicious smoothie to deliver serious protein to your body. The whey protein and milk add up to a whopping 25 grams of protein, which is the perfect amount for your body to absorb at one time. Optimize muscle repair by sipping this within 15 minutes to 1 hour after working out.

- ¾ **cup fat-free milk**
- ½ **ripe banana**
- ½ **cup frozen raspberries**
- ½ **cup frozen blueberries**
- 1 **scoop vanilla whey protein powder**
- 5 **ice cubes**

In a blender, combine all ingredients and puree until smooth.

PER SERVING 285 cal, 27 g pro, 42 g carb, 7 g fiber, 26 g sugars (0 g added sugar), 2 g fat (1 g sat fat), 150 mg sodium

HIGH FIBER   PROTEIN-PACKED

Banana-Almond Protein Smoothie

TOTAL **5 MIN.** // SERVES **1**

If you don't replenish your body after a tough sweat session, you won't see the results from all your hard work. This yummy smoothie delivers 21 grams of protein to help repair microtears in your muscles and get them ready for your next workout.

¼	cup coconut water
¼	cup plain Greek yogurt
1½	Tbsp almond butter
½	scoop whey protein powder
2	tsp hulled hemp seeds
½	frozen banana
½	cup ice

In a blender, combine all ingredients and puree until smooth.

PER SERVING 330 cal, 21 g pro, 26 g carb, 5 g fiber, 15 g sugars (0 g added sugars), 17 g fat (3 g sat fat), 160 mg sodium

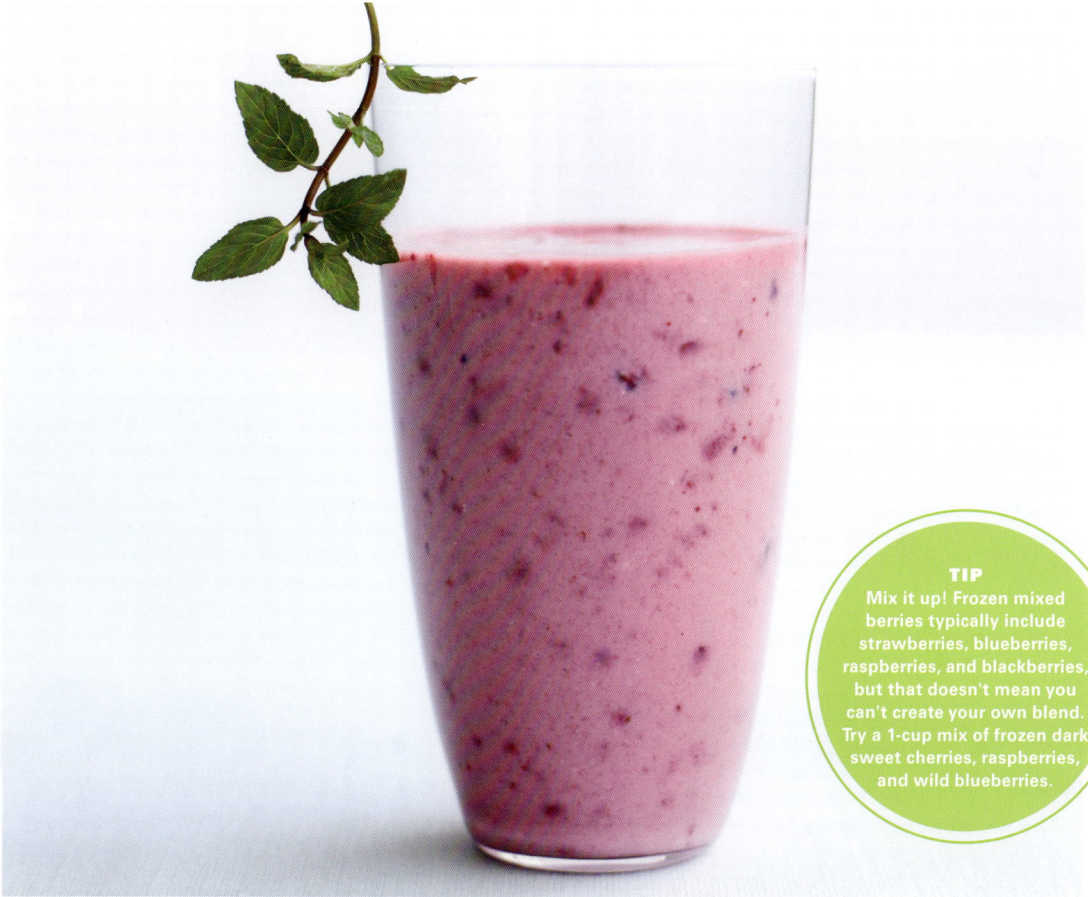

TIP
Mix it up! Frozen mixed berries typically include strawberries, blueberries, raspberries, and blackberries, but that doesn't mean you can't create your own blend. Try a 1-cup mix of frozen dark sweet cherries, raspberries, and wild blueberries.

Pomegranate-Berry Smoothie   **HIGH FIBER**

TOTAL **5 MIN.** // SERVES **1**

Love the tangy-sweet flavor of pomegranate juice? It's time to raise a glass. Research shows that polyphenol-rich pomegranate juice can help fight inflammation related to diseases such as rheumatoid arthritis, inflammatory bowel disease, and metabolic and cardiovascular disorders.

½ **cup chilled pomegranate juice**
½ **cup vanilla low-fat yogurt**
1 **cup frozen mixed berries**

In a blender, combine all ingredients and puree until smooth.

PER SERVING
250 cal, 6 g pro,
52 g carb, 5 g fiber,
44 g sugars
(8 g added sugars),
2 g fat (1 g sat fat),
110 mg sodium

Dishes

TIP
Prepare your jar as directed and refrigerate for up to 2 days. Let sit out at room temperature for at least 10 minutes (this allows the oil to become liquid again) before turning over and dressing.

**VEGETARIAN   HIGH FIBER
PROTEIN-PACKED**

Chickpea Pasta Salad in a Jar

ACTIVE **10 MIN**. // TOTAL **10 MIN**. //
SERVES **1**

This grab-and-go mason jar salad makes eating healthy so easy. Stack your salad the night before (dressing at the bottom lets you avoid soggy lettuce), then toss for a fresh, veggie-packed meal.

¼   **very small onion, finely chopped**
2   **Tbsp red wine vinegar**
2   **Tbsp olive oil**
   Salt and pepper
¼   **cup canned chickpeas, rinsed**
1   **cup grape tomatoes, halved**
2   **Tbsp kalamata olives, halved**
1   **cup cooked spiral pasta**
1½   **cups baby arugula, chopped**
2   **Tbsp crumbled feta**

---

1. In a 1-qt. jar, shake onion, red wine vinegar, oil, and a pinch each salt and pepper. Add chickpeas and gently shake to coat.

2. Top with tomatoes, olives, pasta, arugula, and feta. When ready to serve, turn jar upside down and let sit for 2 min. for the dressing to run over the rest of the ingredients.

PER SERVING 650 cal, 19 g pro, 72 g carb, 11 g fiber, 7 g sugars (0 g added sugars), 31.5 g fat (6.5 g sat fat), 945 mg sodium

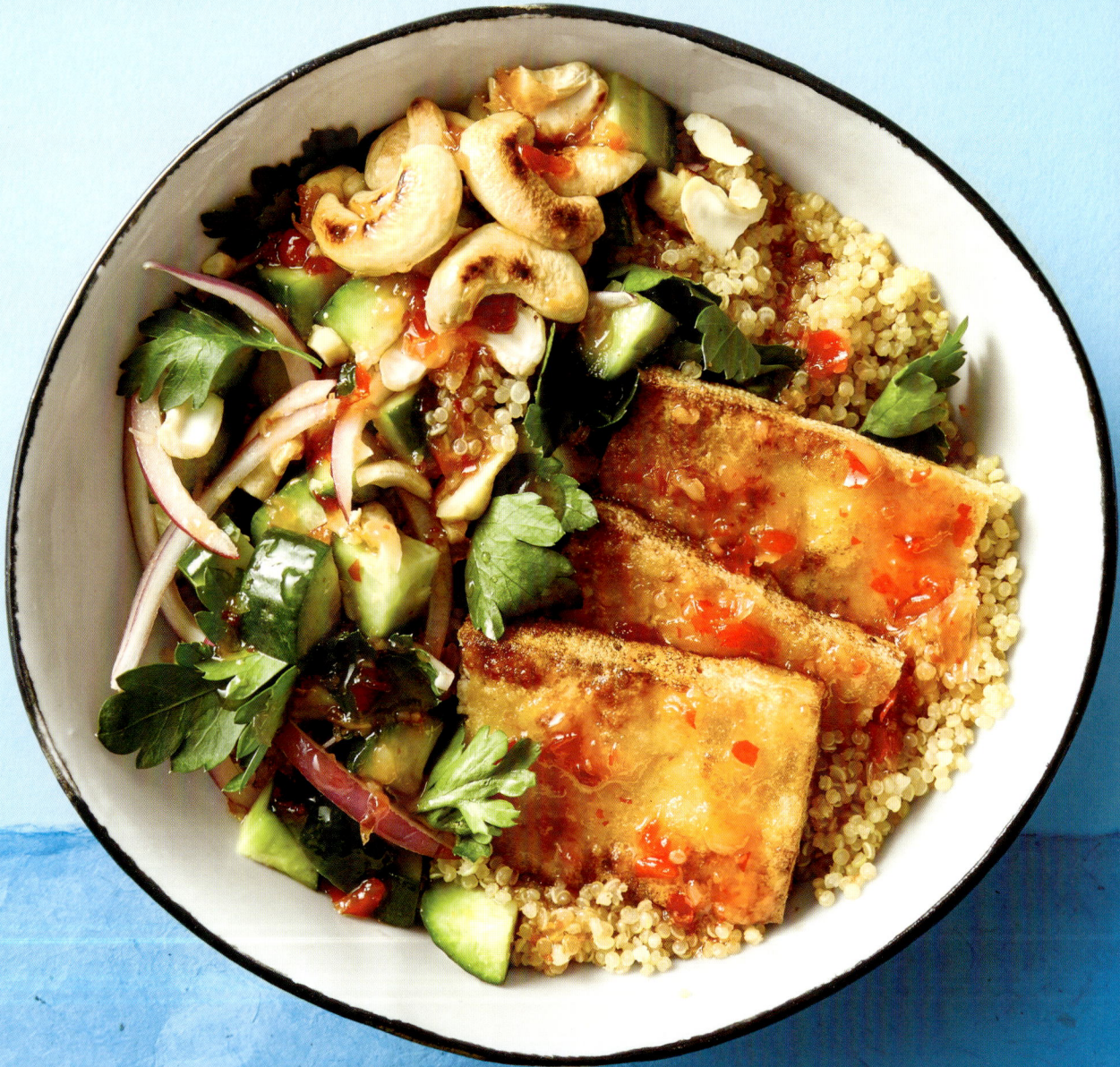

VEGAN HIGH FIBER PROTEIN-PACKED

Crispy Tofu Bowl

ACTIVE **5 MIN**. // TOTAL **30 MIN**. // SERVES **2**

Pan-sautéed tofu adds a delicious crunch to this cucumber-
and cashew-filled vegan quinoa bowl.

1 **14-oz block extra-firm tofu**
¼ **small red onion, very thinly sliced**
2 **Tbsp red wine vinegar**
2 **Tbsp Thai sweet chili sauce**
½ **Tbsp olive oil**
  Kosher salt
½ **seedless cucumber, chopped**
3 **Tbsp cornstarch**
2 **Tbsp canola oil**
½ **cup quinoa, cooked**
1 **Tbsp roasted cashew halves**
  Fresh parsley leaves, for serving

LEFTOVER TIP
Prepare as directed and spoon quinoa into an airtight storage container before topping with cucumber salad, cashews and tofu. Refrigerate quinoa bowl separately from remaining vinaigrette and parsley for up to 2 days. Serve cold or at room temp with drizzled with remaining dressing and topped with parsley leaves.

1. Slice tofu into ¼-in.-thick slices and place them between paper towels on a rimmed baking sheet. Sandwich with a second baking sheet and place a cast-iron skillet or heavy cans on top to weigh it down; press tofu for 10 min. Soak the onion in cold water.

2. In medium bowl, whisk the vinegar, sweet chili sauce, olive oil, and a pinch of salt. Pat the onion dry; toss with half of the vinaigrette and the cucumber.

3. Sprinkle tofu on both sides with cornstarch. Heat canola oil in a large pan on medium-high until hot. Carefully add the tofu and cook until deep golden brown, 2 to 3 min. per side. Drain on paper towels.

4. Divide quinoa between two bowls. Top with cucumber salad, cashews, parsley, and tofu. Drizzle with remaining vinaigrette.

PER SERVING
565 cal, 28 g pro, 57 g carb, 7 g fiber, 13 g sugars (10 g added sugars), 25 g fat (3 g sat fat), 175 mg sodium

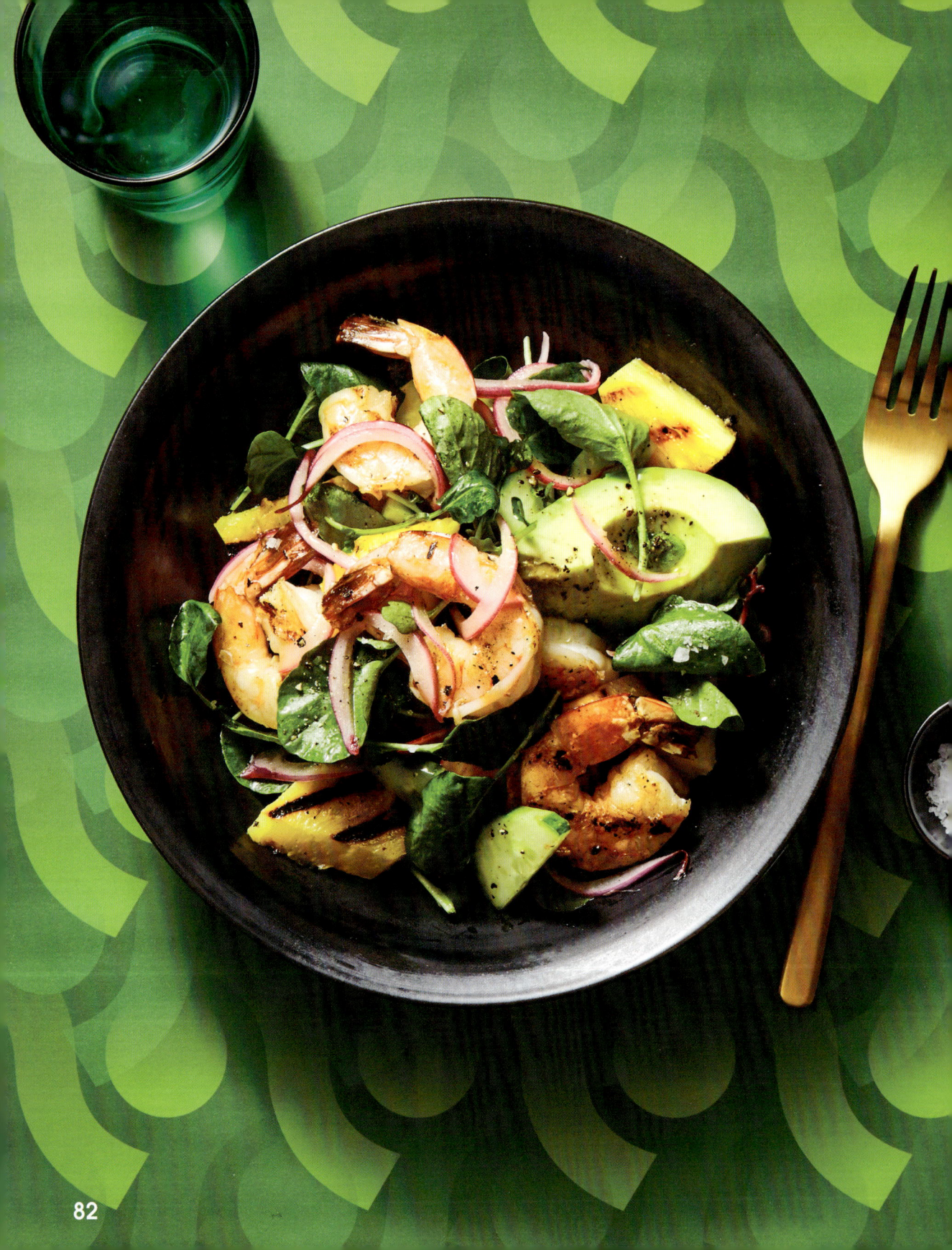

HIGH FIBER PROTEIN-PACKED

Charred Shrimp and Avocado Salad

ACTIVE **10 MIN.** // TOTAL **25 MIN.** // SERVES **2**

Shrimp are quick cooking and packed with protein, making them a great alternative to the usual lean chicken breast when you're trying to eat healthy.

½   lb large shrimp, peeled and deveined

2   Tbsp plus 1 tsp olive oil, divided
Kosher salt and pepper

2   ½-in.-thick slices pineapple, rind discarded

1   Tbsp fresh lemon juice

¼   small red onion, thinly sliced

1   Persian cucumber, sliced into half-moons

½   bunch upland watercress

½   avocado, cut into wedges

1. Heat grill pan or grill on medium high or heat broiler. Toss shrimp with 1 Tbsp oil and ¼ tsp each salt and pepper. Brush pineapple with 1 tsp oil. Grill or broil until pineapple is slightly charred and shrimp are opaque throughout, about 3 min. per side on the grill or 6 to 8 min. in broiler (rotating pan and turning food over halfway through).

2. Meanwhile, in bowl, whisk together lemon juice, remaining Tbsp oil and pinch each salt and pepper. Toss with onion.

3. Cut grilled pineapple into smaller pieces. Add to bowl with onion along with cucumber and shrimp and toss to combine. Fold in watercress and avocado.

PER SERVING
355 cal, 18 g pro, 18 g carb, 5 g fiber, 9 g sugars (0 g added sugars), 25 g fat (3.5 g sat fat), 950 mg sodium

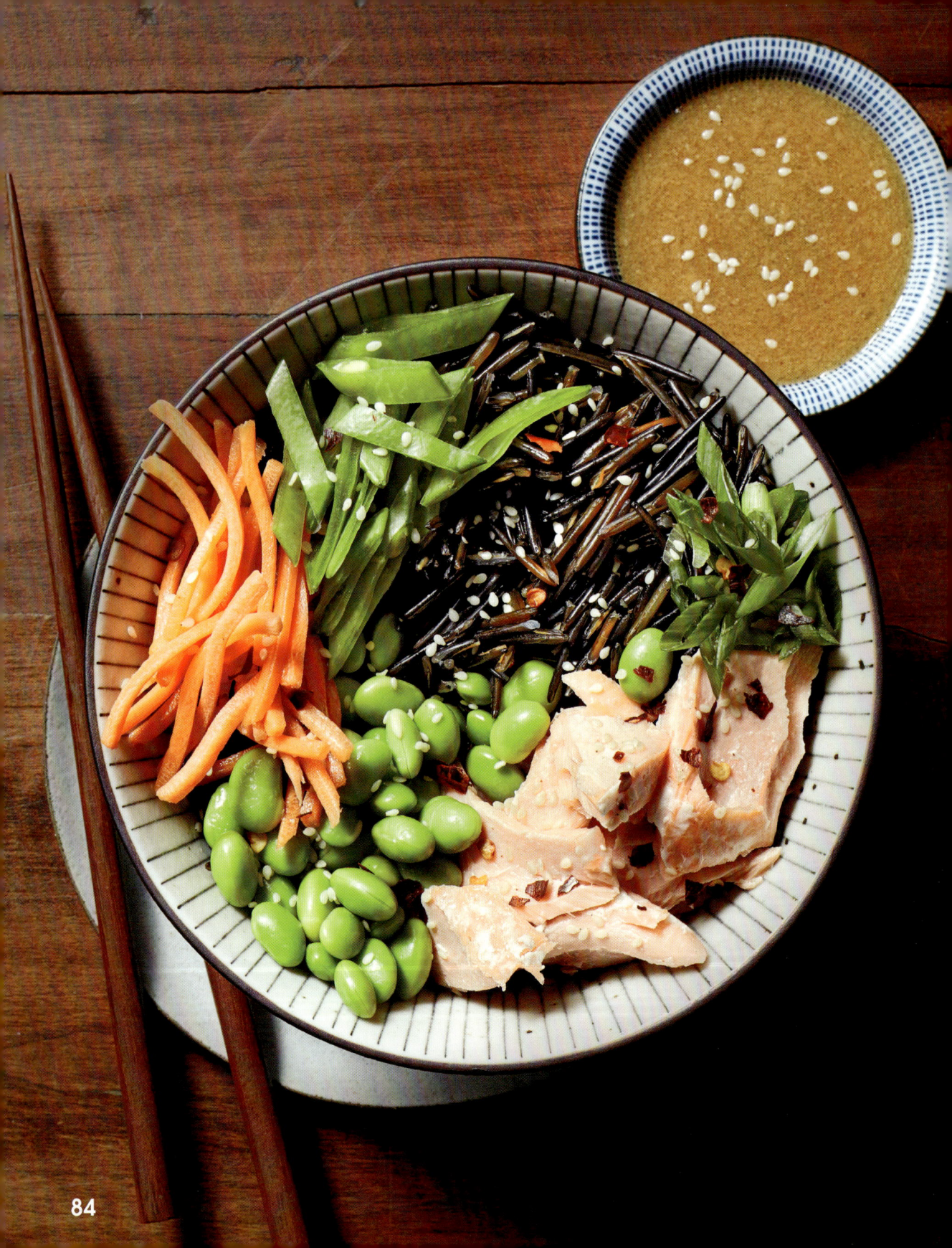

HIGH FIBER PROTEIN-PACKED
Asian Salmon Bowl

ACTIVE **10 MIN**. // TOTAL **1 HR 5 MIN**. // SERVES **2**

This dish has all the Chinese takeout flavor you crave for
a fraction of the calories and sodium.

- 4   tsp rice vinegar
- 1   Tbsp miso paste
- 2   tsp less-sodium soy sauce
- ½   tsp grated fresh ginger
- 2   Tbsp vegetable oil
- 2   tsp toasted sesame oil
- 1½ cups cooked wild rice
- 1   6-oz can salmon, drained
- ½   cup frozen shelled edamame, thawed
- ½   cup shredded carrots
- ½   cup snow peas
- 1   large scallion, sliced
- ½   tsp sesame seeds
-     Red pepper flakes, for garnish

1. Whisk together the vinegar, miso, soy sauce, ginger, oils, and 1 Tbsp warm water.

2. Divide rice between 2 bowls and top each with salmon, edamame, carrots, and snow peas.

3. Drizzle with dressing and top with scallion and sesame seeds.

4. Garnish with red pepper flakes.

PER SERVING
495 cal, 26 g pro,
47 g carb, 7 g
fiber, 6 g sugars
(0 g added
sugars), 23 g fat
(3 g sat fat),
720 mg sodium

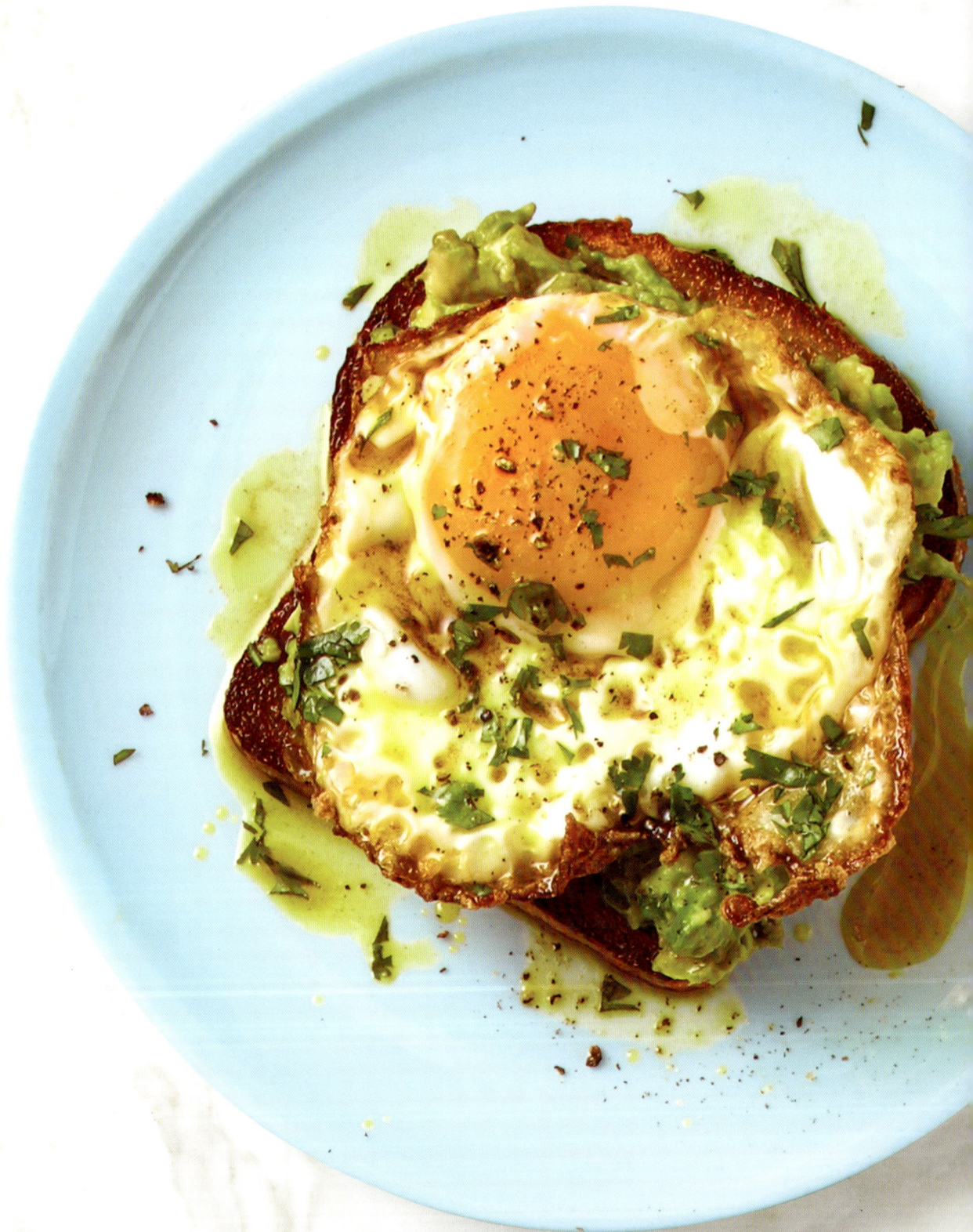

VEGETARIAN HIGH FIBER

Curry-Avocado Crispy Egg Toast

ACTIVE **10 MIN**. // TOTAL **10 MIN**. // SERVES **1**

Start your day with this flavorful dish. The turmeric in curry powder provides an antioxidant and anti-inflammatory boost.

¼   **tsp curry powder**

1½ **Tbsp olive oil, divided**

¼   **large avocado**

1   **tsp fresh lime juice**
    Kosher salt and pepper

1   **slice whole-grain bread, toasted**

1   **large egg**
    Finely chopped cilantro

1. In a small dry skillet on medium, toast curry powder until fragrant, 1 min. Stir in 1 Tbsp olive oil and set aside.

2. Mash avocado with lime juice and pinch salt and spread on toast.

3. In medium nonstick skillet on medium-high, heat remaining ½ Tbsp oil. Add egg and cook until whites are golden brown, crisp around edges, and yolk is desired doneness, about 2 min. for runny yolks (if edges are dark but whites are not set, remove skillet from heat; cover until whites are cooked, about 10 seconds). Season with pinch each salt and pepper.

4. Top each slice of avocado toast with egg and chopped cilantro, then drizzle with curry oil.

PER SERVING
450 cal, 13 g pro, 24 g carb, 8 g fiber, 4 g sugars (0 g added sugars), 34.5 g fat (6 g sat fat), 380 mg sodium

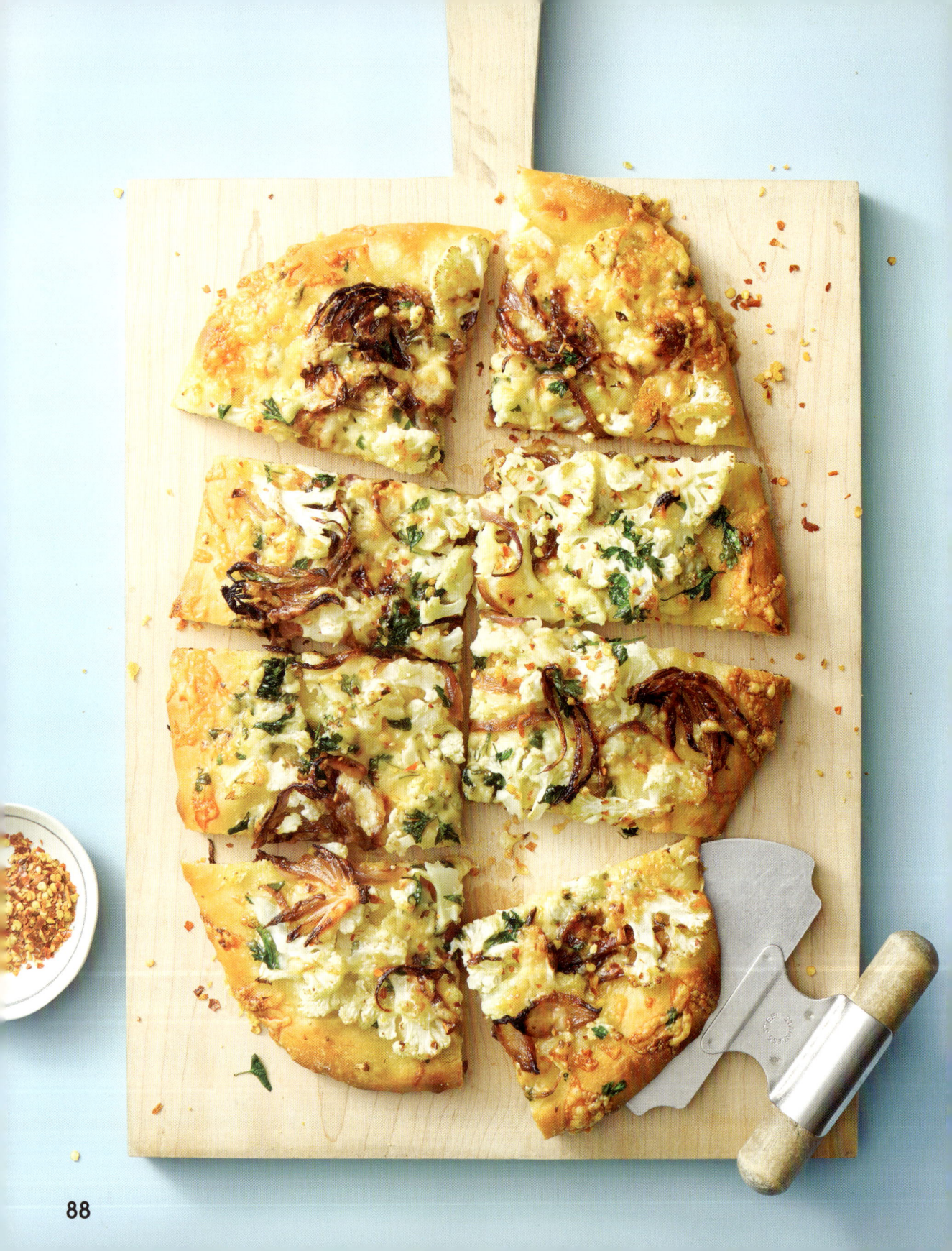

VEGETARIAN PROTEIN-PACKED
Roasted Cauliflower Pizza

ACTIVE **10 MIN**. // TOTAL **40 MIN**. // SERVES **4**

Given cauliflower's low caloric content, it's a great choice for those trying to lose weight. You can substantially cut down on calories and carbohydrates when choosing cauliflower, while adding in extra fiber to help keep you full. And the best way to enjoy it: putting it on pizza!

Cornmeal

1 **lb pizza dough**

½ **medium head (about 1 lb) cauliflower, thinly sliced**

1 **small red onion, thinly sliced**

½ **cup fresh flat-leaf parsley**

2 **Tbsp olive oil**

¼ **tsp crushed red pepper, optional**

½ **tsp salt**

4 **oz (about 1¾ cups) Gruyère cheese, coarsely grated**

1. Heat oven to 425°F. Dust baking sheet with cornmeal. Shape pizza dough into 16-in. oval and place on prepared sheet.

2. In large bowl, toss cauliflower, red onion, and fresh flat-leaf parsley leaves with olive oil, crushed red pepper (optional), and salt. Fold in Gruyère cheese.

3. Scatter vegetable mixture over dough. Bake until cauliflower is tender and crust is golden brown and crisp, 20 to 25 min.

PER SERVING
335 cal, 15 g pro, 32 g carb, 2 g fiber, 3 g sugars (0 g added sugars), 16 g fat (6 g sat fat), 740 mg sodium

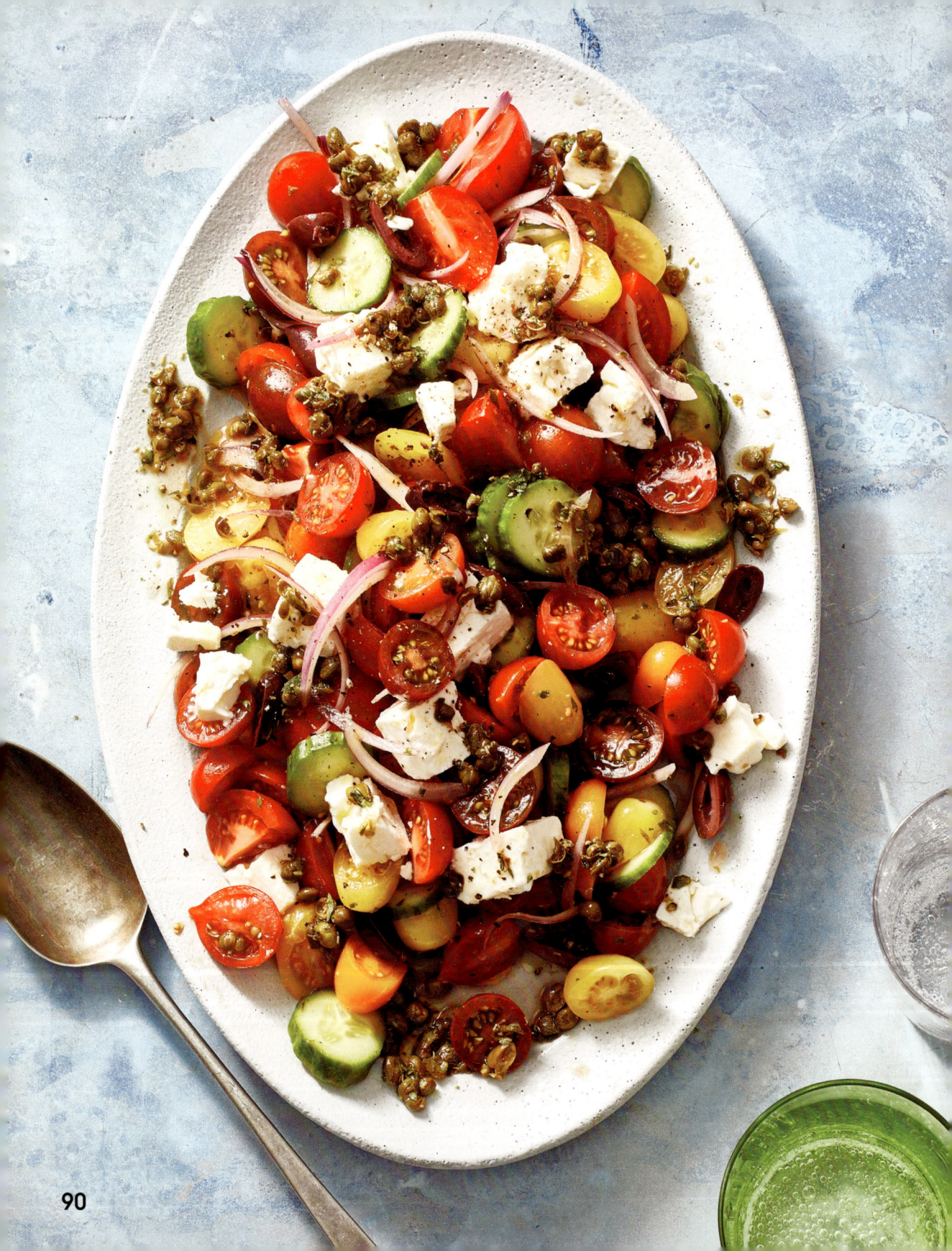

VEGETARIAN
Greek Salad

ACTIVE **20 MIN.** // TOTAL **20 MIN.** // SERVES **2**

Try this delicious and healthy Greek salad recipe, which brings an easy staple of Mediterranean cuisine to your home. Briny capers give this crowd favorite a secret boost of flavor and they're packed with antioxidants that help reduce inflammation.

1½ Tbsp red wine vinegar

1 Tbsp olive oil

1 tsp confectioners' sugar
Kosher salt and pepper

1 Tbsp capers, drained and roughly chopped

½ tsp fresh oregano, chopped

½ lb mixed cherry, grape, and campari tomatoes, halved or cut into wedges

4 oz Persian cucumbers, cut into ¼-in.-thick rounds

¼ very small red onion, thinly sliced

2 Tbsp pitted Kalamata olives, halved
Feta cheese, cut into small cubes, for serving

1. In small bowl, whisk together vinegar, oil, sugar, and pinch each salt and pepper. Stir in capers and oregano.

2. Arrange tomatoes and cucumbers on a platter and scatter onion and olives on top. Spoon dressing over salad and serve with feta if desired.

PER SERVING
120 cal, 2 g pro, 9 g carb, 2 g fiber, 4 g sugars (1 g added sugars), 9 g fat (1.5 g sat fat), 295 mg sodium

LEFTOVER TIP
Refrigerate leftovers in an airtight container for up to 2 days.

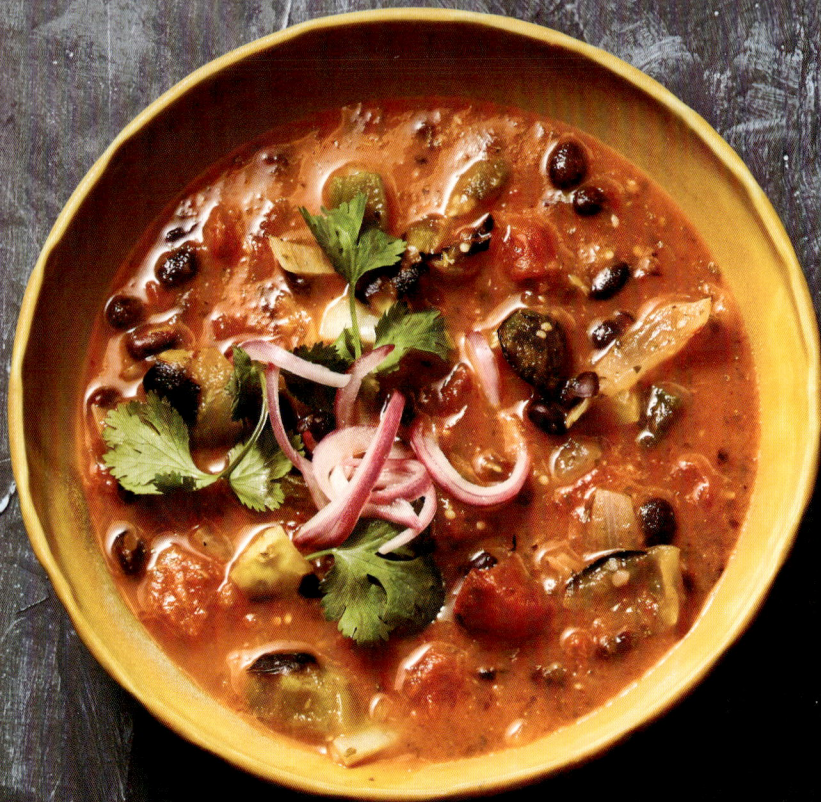
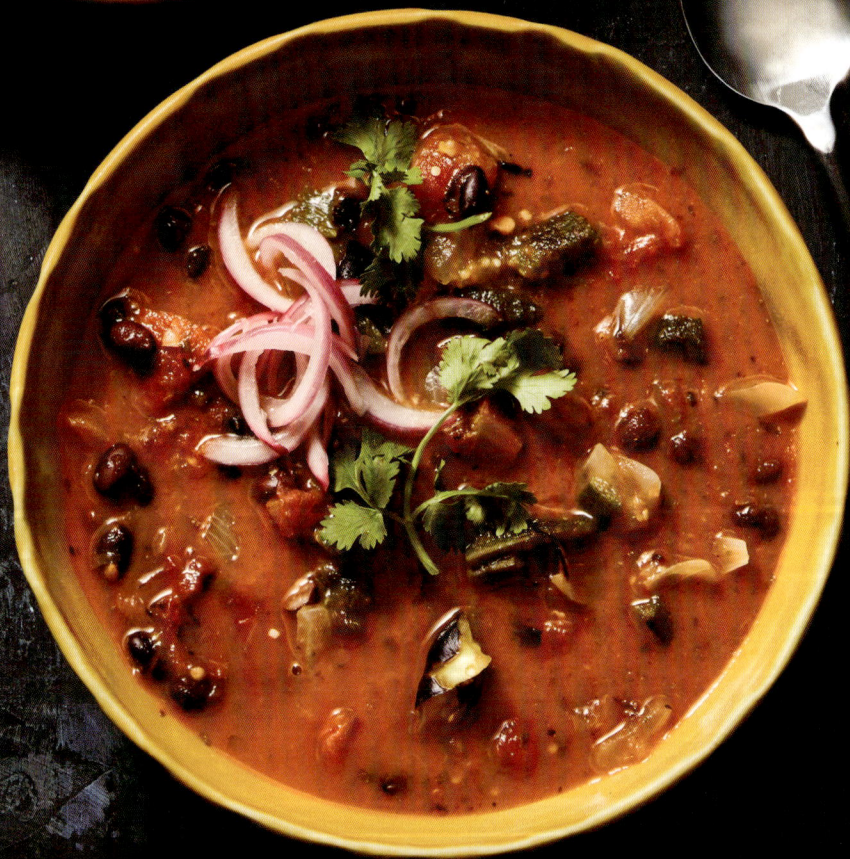

VEGETARIAN HIGH FIBER PROTEIN-PACKED

Fiery Black Bean Soup

ACTIVE **10 MIN.** // TOTAL **45 MIN.** // SERVES **4**

Warm up with this cozy bowl. It's not just good for the soul; the capsaicin, a compound that makes peppers hot, may also give you a quick metabolism boost.

8	oz tomatillos (about 4), husks removed, halved
2	cloves garlic, unpeeled
1	large yellow onion, cut into 1-in.-thick wedges
1	large poblano pepper, halved and seeded
1	jalapeño, halved and seeded
1	Tbsp olive oil
	Kosher salt and pepper
½	tsp ground cumin
½	tsp ground coriander
4	cups low-sodium chicken broth
2	15-oz cans low-sodium black beans, rinsed
1	14.5-oz can fire-roasted diced tomatoes, drained
1	small red onion, thinly sliced
2	Tbsp fresh lime juice
	Cilantro leaves, for serving

1. Heat broiler. On large rimmed baking sheet, toss tomatillos, garlic, yellow onion, poblano, and jalapeño with oil and ½ tsp each salt and pepper. Turn peppers cut-side down and broil, rotating pan every 5 min., until vegetables are tender and charred, 15 min.

2. Discard skins from poblanos and garlic. Finely chop vegetables and transfer to Dutch oven. Add cumin and coriander and cook on medium, stirring occasionally, 2 min. Add broth, beans, and tomatoes and bring to a simmer; cook 4 min.

3. Meanwhile, toss red onion with lime juice and a pinch each of salt and pepper; let sit at least 10 min. Serve soup topped with pickled onions and cilantro.

PER SERVING
325 cal, 20 g pro, 53 g carb, 18 g fiber, 8 g sugars (0 g added sugars), 6 g fat (1 g sat fat), 705 mg sodium

TIP
Leftovers can be refrigerated in an airtight container for up to 5 days or frozen for up to 3 months.

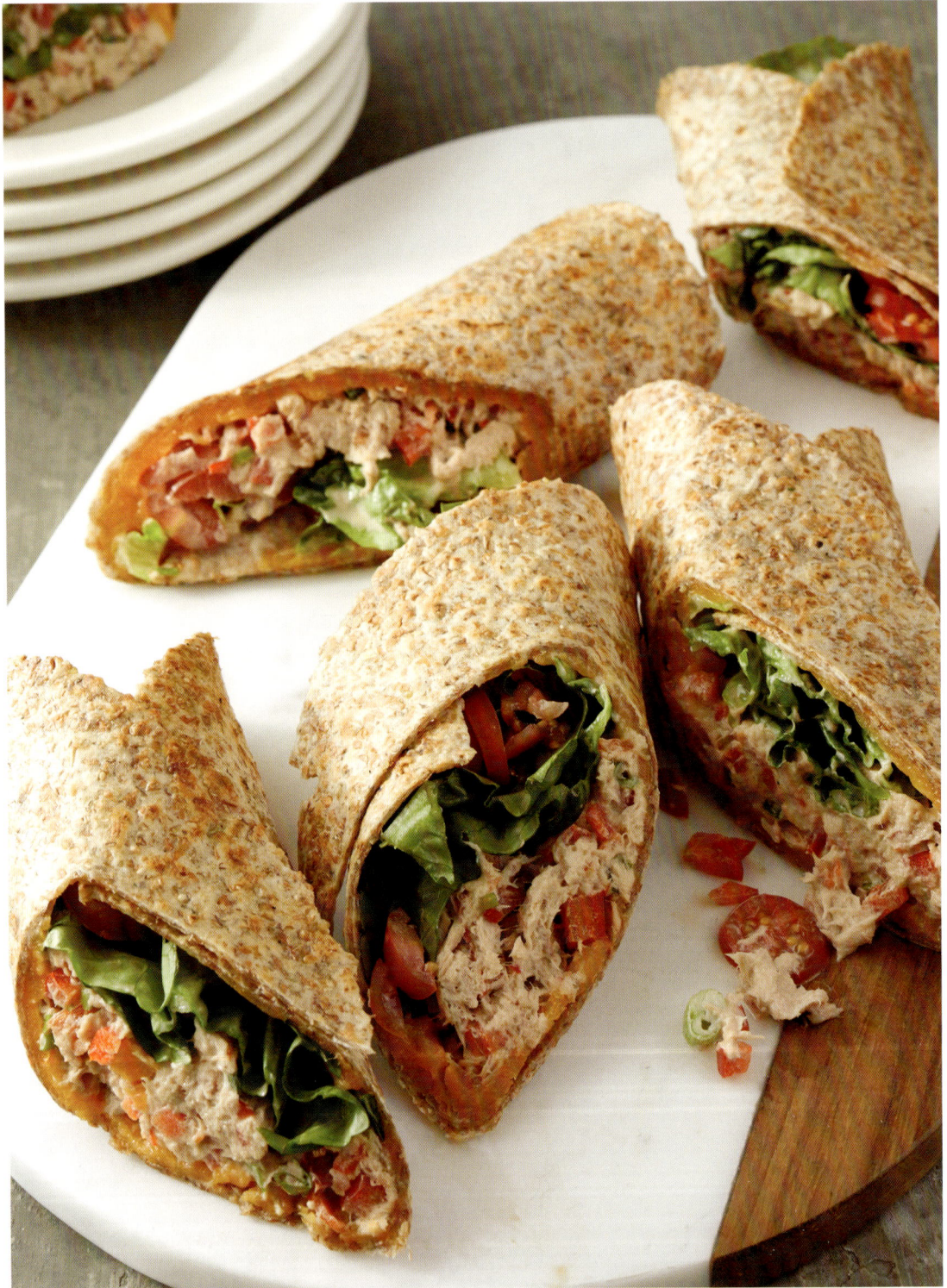

HIGH FIBER **PROTEIN-PACKED**
Tuna and Cheddar Wraps

ACTIVE **10 MIN**. // TOTAL **10 MIN**. // SERVES **1**

If you're truly strapped for time and need a nutrient-dense recipe ASAP, this is one to memorize. These low-fat portable wraps take just 10 minutes to put together and provide a whopping 32 grams of protein and 5 grams of fiber.

- 1 **3-oz pouch tuna fish**
- 1 **Tbsp olive oil mayonnaise**
- ½ **scallion, finely chopped**
- ¼ **red pepper, finely chopped**
- 1 **tsp olive oil**
- 1 **8-inch whole-grain tortilla**
- 1 **oz sharp Cheddar, coarsely grated**
- 2 **pieces butter lettuce**
- ½ **cup grape tomatoes, sliced**

1. In a large bowl, combine tuna, mayo, scallions, and red pepper.

2. In a large nonstick skillet on medium, heat 1 tsp oil. Cook tortilla until beginning to brown, 1 min. Flip, top with cheese, and cook until cheese is melted. Transfer to plate.

3. Spread tuna mixture down center of tortilla, then top with lettuce and tomatoes and roll up.

PER SERVING
485 cal, 32 g pro,
32 g carb, 5 g fiber,
3 g sugar
(0 g added sugars),
27 g fat (8.5 g
sat fat), 960 mg
sodium

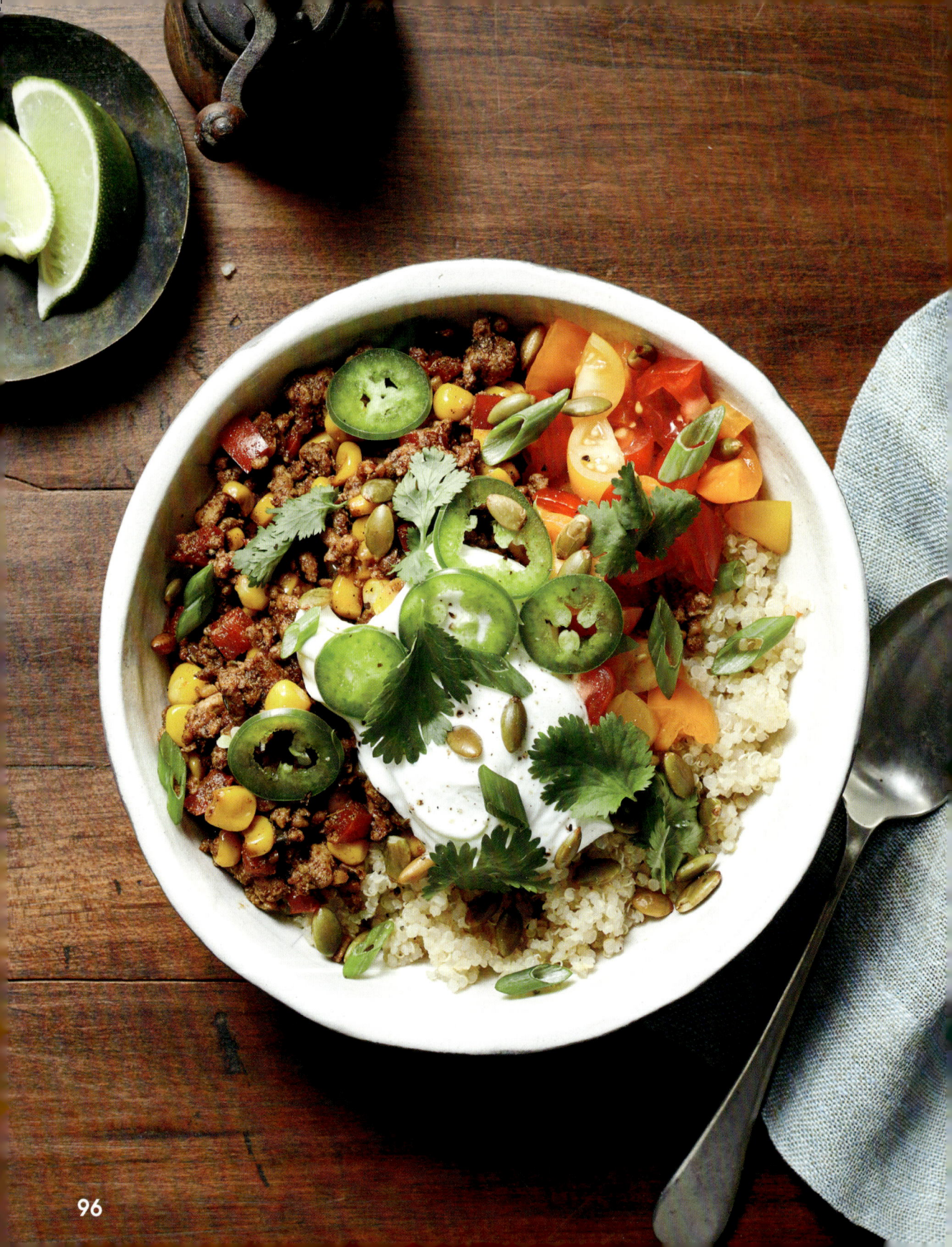

HIGH FIBER PROTEIN-PACKED

Loaded Taco Bowl

ACTIVE **10 MIN**. // TOTAL **35 MIN**. // SERVES **2**

By ditching the tortillas in favor of quinoa and swapping beef for turkey, this bowl cuts your intake of refined carbs and saturated fat while delivering 34 grams of filling protein.

1	Tbsp vegetable oil
2	large scallions, sliced (white and green parts)
1	clove garlic, minced
½	red bell pepper, diced
½	lb lean ground turkey
½	cup frozen corn kernels
4	tsp chili powder
2	tsp ground cumin
½	tsp kosher salt
½	tsp black pepper
1	cup cooked quinoa
½	cup halved cherry tomatoes
¼	cup cilantro
¼	cup fat-free Greek yogurt
2	Tbsp pepitas
½	jalapeno, sliced
	Lime wedges, for serving

1. Heat oil over medium-high in a large skillet.

2. Cook white parts of scallions, garlic, and bell pepper until soft, 4 min.

3. Add turkey and cook until browned and cooked through, 5 min. Stir in corn, chili powder, cumin, salt, and pepper.

4. Remove from heat.

5. Divide quinoa between 2 bowls and top with turkey mixture and remaining ingredients.

6. Serve with lime wedges.

PER SERVING
475 cal, 34 g pro, 42 g carb, 6 g fiber, 6 g sugars (0 g added sugars), 20.5 g fat (4 g sat fat), 605 mg sodium

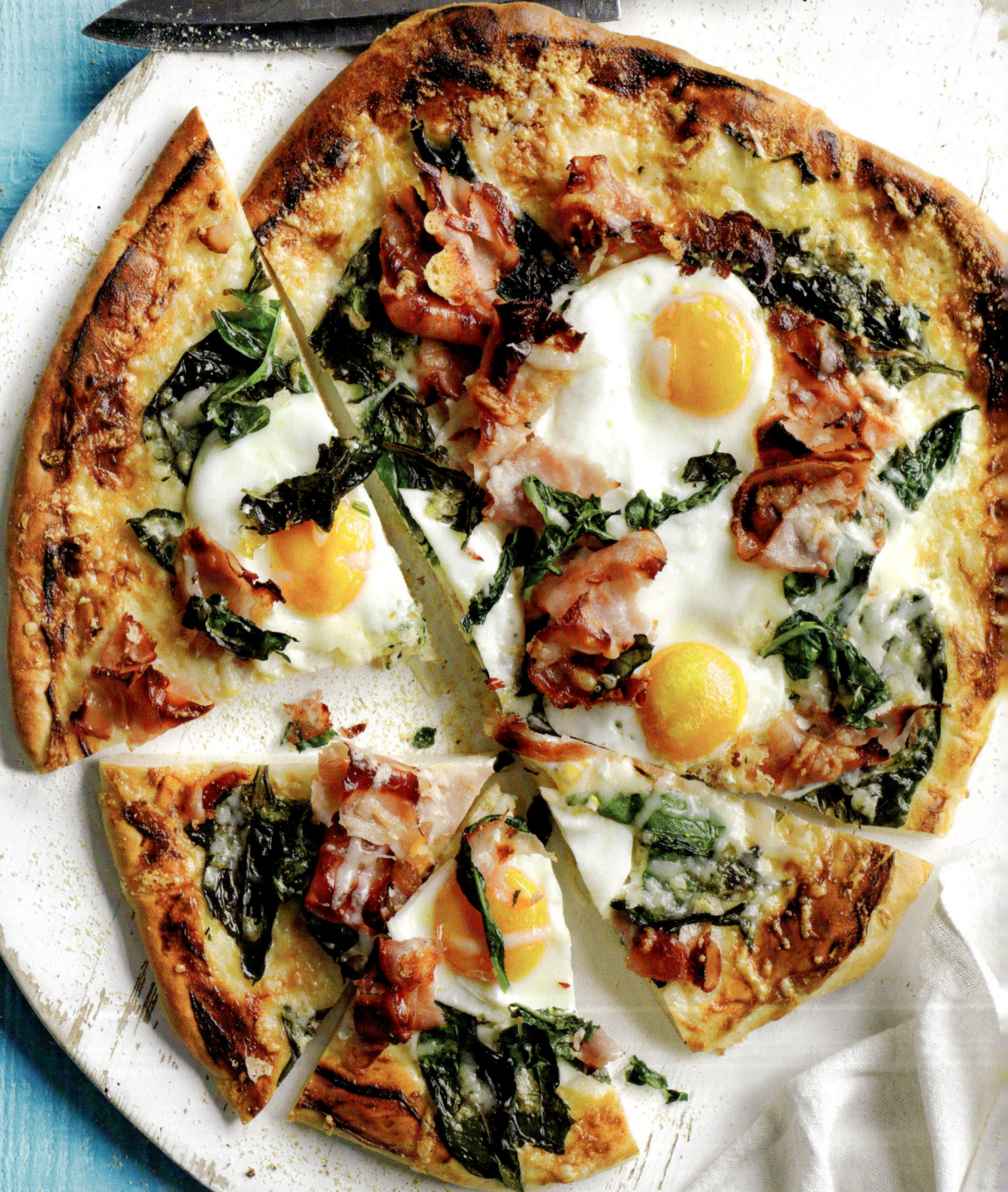

PROTEIN-PACKED
Sunny-Side-Up Pizza

ACTIVE **10 MIN**. // TOTAL **25 MIN**. // SERVES **4**

Indulge for less than 500 calories a serving when you prepare this healthy, fit-for-brunch pizza. You've never had bacon, egg, and cheese like this before.

Cornmeal, for baking sheet
Flour, for surface

1   lb pizza dough, thawed if frozen
1   Tbsp Dijon mustard
2   oz Gruyère cheese, coarsely grated (about ½ cup), divided
2   oz deli ham, thinly sliced
1   bunch spinach, thick stems discarded
4   large eggs
    Green salad, for serving

1. Heat oven to 450°F. Lightly dust baking sheet with cornmeal. On floured surface, shape dough into 16-in. circle. Place on prepared sheet.

2. Spread mustard over dough, then sprinkle with three-fourths of the Gruyère. Top with ham, spinach, and remaining Gruyère.

3. Working with 1 egg at a time, crack eggs into small bowl, then slide onto pizza. Bake until egg whites are set and crust is golden brown, 15 to 17 min. Serve with salad if desired.

PER SERVING
(¼ of the pie)
450 cal, 22 g pro,
55 g carb, 2 g fiber,
3 g sugars (2 g
added sugars),
15 g fat (6.5 g
sat fat), 755 mg
sodium

LEFTOVER TIP
If you're eating only 2 slices, use 2 eggs and position them on one half to eat immediately. Save the remaining pizza for up to a week, then reheat and top with a sunny-side-up egg.

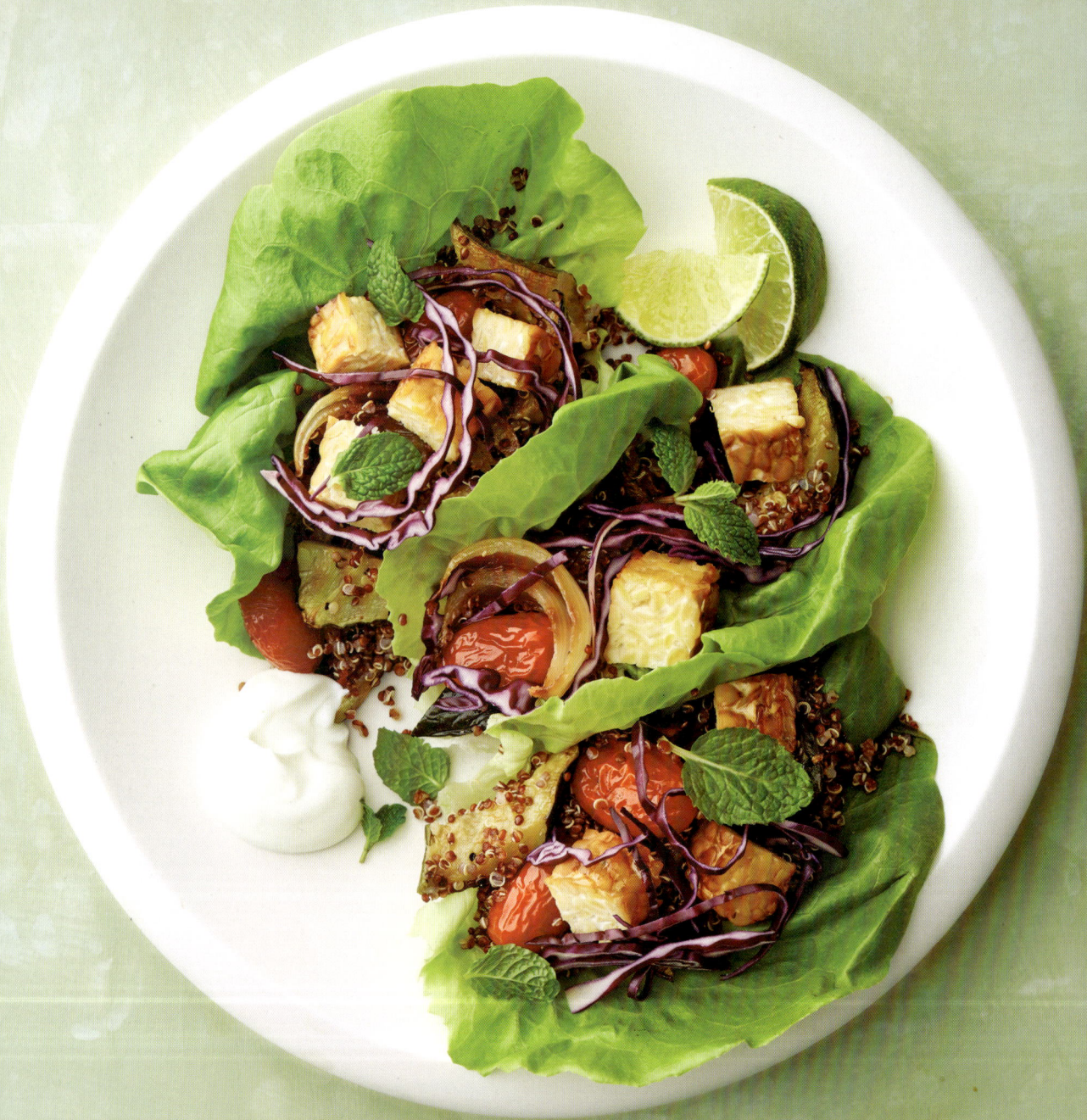

VEGETARIAN   HIGH FIBER   PROTEIN-PACKED

Easy Tempeh Lettuce Wraps

ACTIVE **10 MIN.** // TOTAL **20 MIN.** // SERVES **2**

Tempeh is high in protein and has a texture that is close to meat, so it makes a great substitute. Try it with this delicious vegetarian recipe—it's filling, with a whopping 20 grams of protein, and takes only 20 minutes to whip up!

½ **cup quinoa**

½ **small zucchini, cut into 1-inch pieces**

½ **small onion, sliced**

½ **cup grape tomatoes**

½ **Tbsp olive oil**

Kosher salt and pepper

4 **oz roasted tempeh, cut into pieces**

½ **cup shredded red cabbage**

½ **head Boston lettuce**

Greek yogurt, mint leaves and lime wedges, for serving

1. Heat oven to 450°F. Cook quinoa per package directions.

2. On rimmed baking sheet, toss zucchini, onion, and tomatoes with oil, and season with ¼ tsp each salt and pepper. Roast until just tender, 10 to 12 min.; transfer to bowl.

3. Fluff quinoa and add to bowl with vegetables along with tempeh and red cabbage; toss to combine.

4. Separate leaves from lettuce head. Fill lettuce leaves with quinoa mixture and top with mint leaves. Dollop with Greek yogurt and serve with lime wedges.

PER SERVING
340 cal, 20 g pro,
41 g carb, 9 g fiber,
5 g sugars
(0 g added sugars),
13 g fat (2.5 g
sat fat), 270 mg
sodium

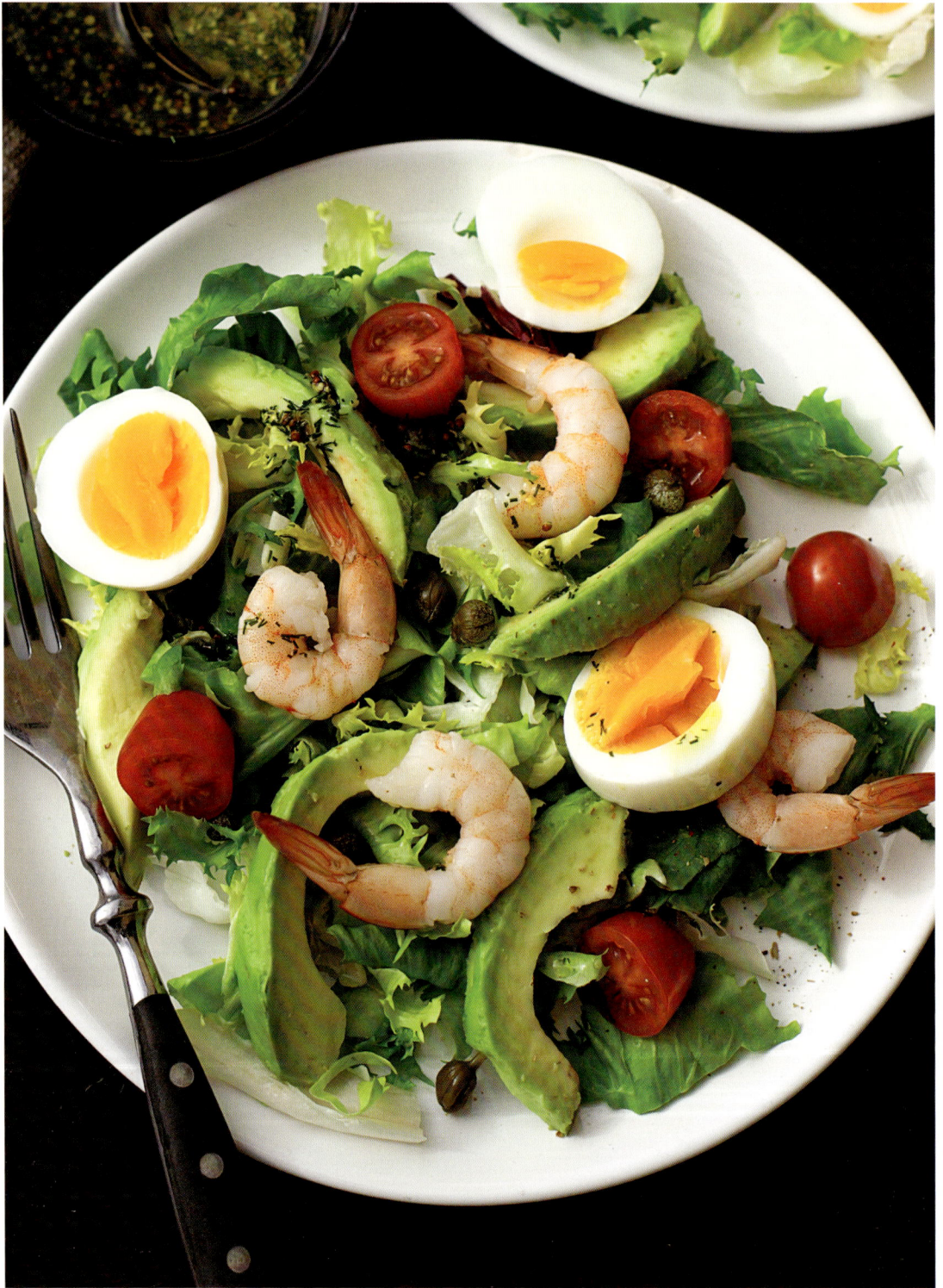

HIGH FIBER PROTEIN-PACKED

Shrimp, Avocado, and Egg Chopped Salad

ACTIVE **10 MIN**. // TOTAL **15 MIN**. // SERVES **1**

Shrimp is high in protein and low in calories, making it an ideal alternative to beef and chicken. Paired with some pre-made hard-boiled eggs and nutrient-dense veggies, this chopped salad recipe boasts 41 grams of filling protein per serving.

⅛ small red onion, thinly sliced
1 Tbsp fresh lime juice
½ Tbsp olive oil, divided
6 oz large shrimp, peeled and deveined
  Kosher salt and pepper
½ cup grape tomatoes, halved
4 cups butter lettuce
¼ cup fresh cilantro leaves
¼ avocado, diced
1 hard-boiled egg, cut into pieces

1. In a large bowl, toss onion with lime juice and ¼ Tbsp oil and let sit for 5 min.

2. In a large skillet on medium-high, heat ¼ Tbsp oil. Season shrimp with ¼ tsp each salt and pepper and cook until opaque throughout, 1 to 2 min. per side.

3. Toss tomatoes with onion, then toss with lettuce and cilantro. Spoon into a bowl and top with shrimp, avocado, and egg.

PER SERVING
395 cal, 41 g pro, 19 g carb, 7 g fiber, 5 g sugars (0 g added sugars), 21 g fat (4 g sat fat), 750 mg sodium

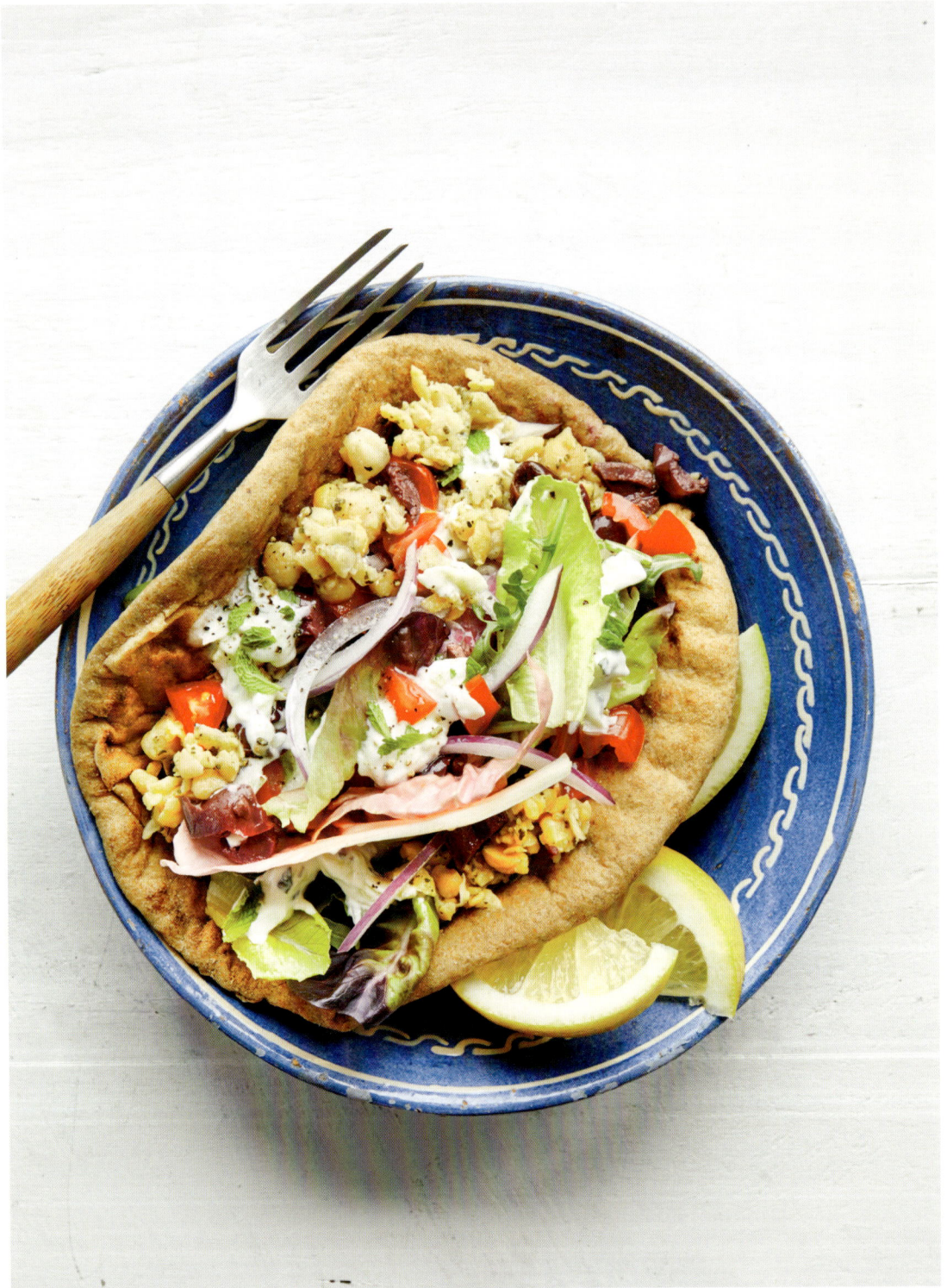

VEGETARIAN HIGH FIBER PROTEIN-PACKED

Greek Chickpea Tacos

ACTIVE **10 MIN**. // TOTAL **20 MIN**. // SERVES **2**

These low-calorie tacos look and taste like summer on a plate! With tons of bright veggies and homemade tzatziki sauce, these vegetarian pitas make eating healthy so much more fun.

½ **cup canned low-sodium chickpeas, rinsed**

1 **Tbsp olive oil**

½ **tsp dried oregano**

1 **Tbsp fresh lemon juice, divided**
   Kosher salt and pepper

2 **whole-wheat pitas, warmed**

1 **cup mixed greens**

1 **plum tomato, cut into ¼-in. pieces**

¼ **small red onion, thinly sliced**

2 **Tbsp pitted kalamata olives, sliced**

1 **Persian cucumber, grated (reserve and dice extra cucumber for garnish, if desired)**

½ **cup plain Greek yogurt**

½ **clove garlic, grated**

1 **Tbsp chopped fresh mint and whole leaves for serving**

1. In a medium bowl, mash chickpeas with oil, then add oregano, ½ Tbsp lemon juice and pinch each salt and pepper. Spread half onto each pita. Top with greens, tomato, onion, and olives.

2. In a medium bowl, combine cucumber, yogurt, garlic, remaining ½ Tbsp lemon juice, pinch salt, and chopped mint. Spoon over pitas and top with mint leaves and chopped cucumber, if desired.

PER SERVING
385 cal, 16 g pro, 53 g carb, 8 g fiber, 8 g sugars (0 g added sugars), 12 g fat (3 g sat fat), 585 mg sodium

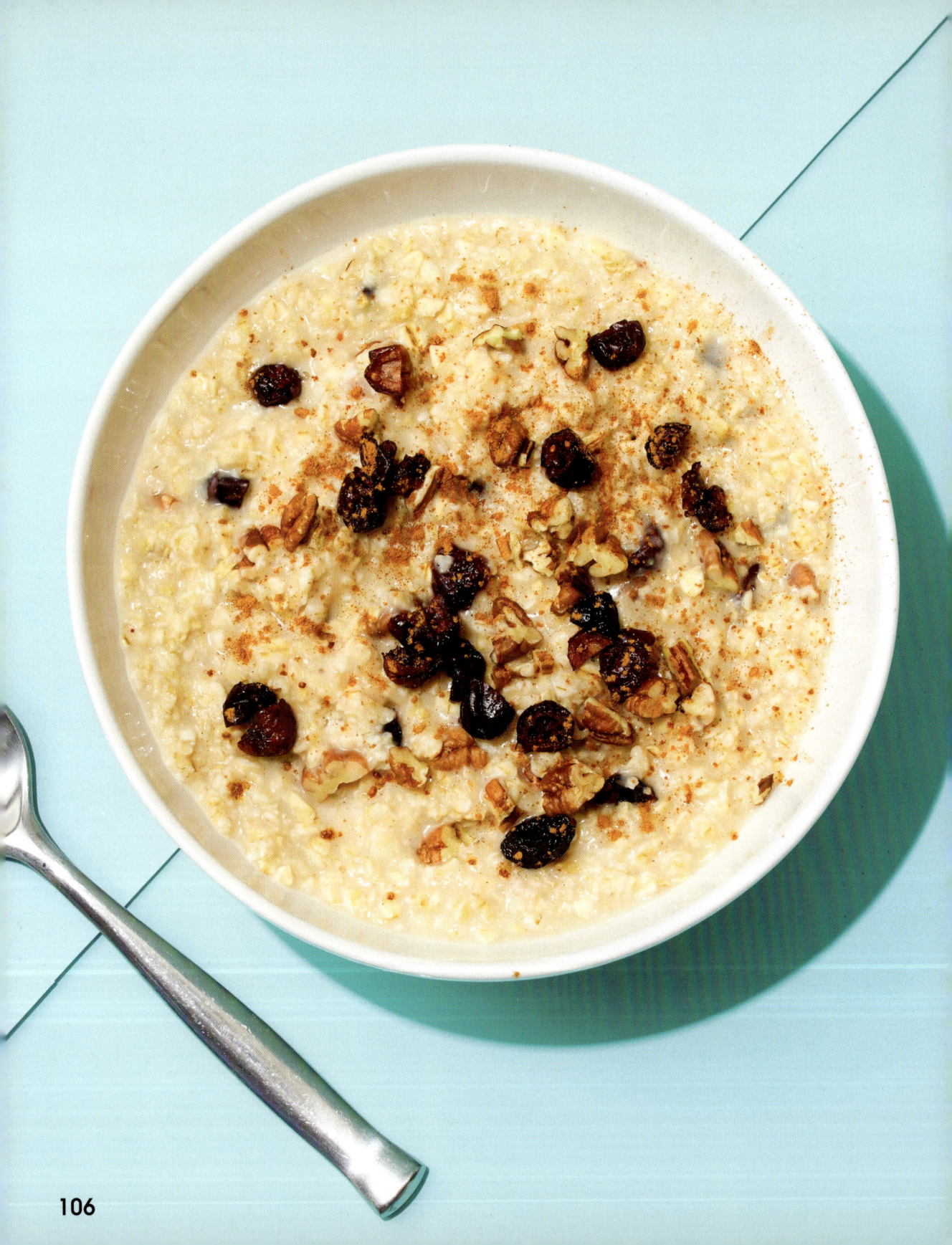

HIGH FIBER

Instant Oatmeal with Cranberries and Pecans

ACTIVE **5 MIN.** // TOTAL **5 MIN.** // SERVES **1**

Get fresher flavors with this quick, healthy breakfast recipe that you can make from scratch rather than relying on store-bought.

¼ **cup quick oats**
1 **Tbsp dried cranberries**
1 **Tbsp chopped toasted pecans**
½ **tsp brown sugar**
Ground cinnamon
Grated orange zest
Kosher salt

1. In medium bowl, place quick oats, cranberries, pecans, and brown sugar, plus pinch each of ground cinnamon, grated orange zest, and salt.

2. Add ½ to ¾ cup just-boiling water. Let sit 1 min. Stir and eat.

PER SERVING
190 cal, 4 g pro,
32 g carb, 6 g fiber,
10 g sugars
(6 g added sugars),
6.5 g fat
(0.5 g sat fat),
120 mg sodium

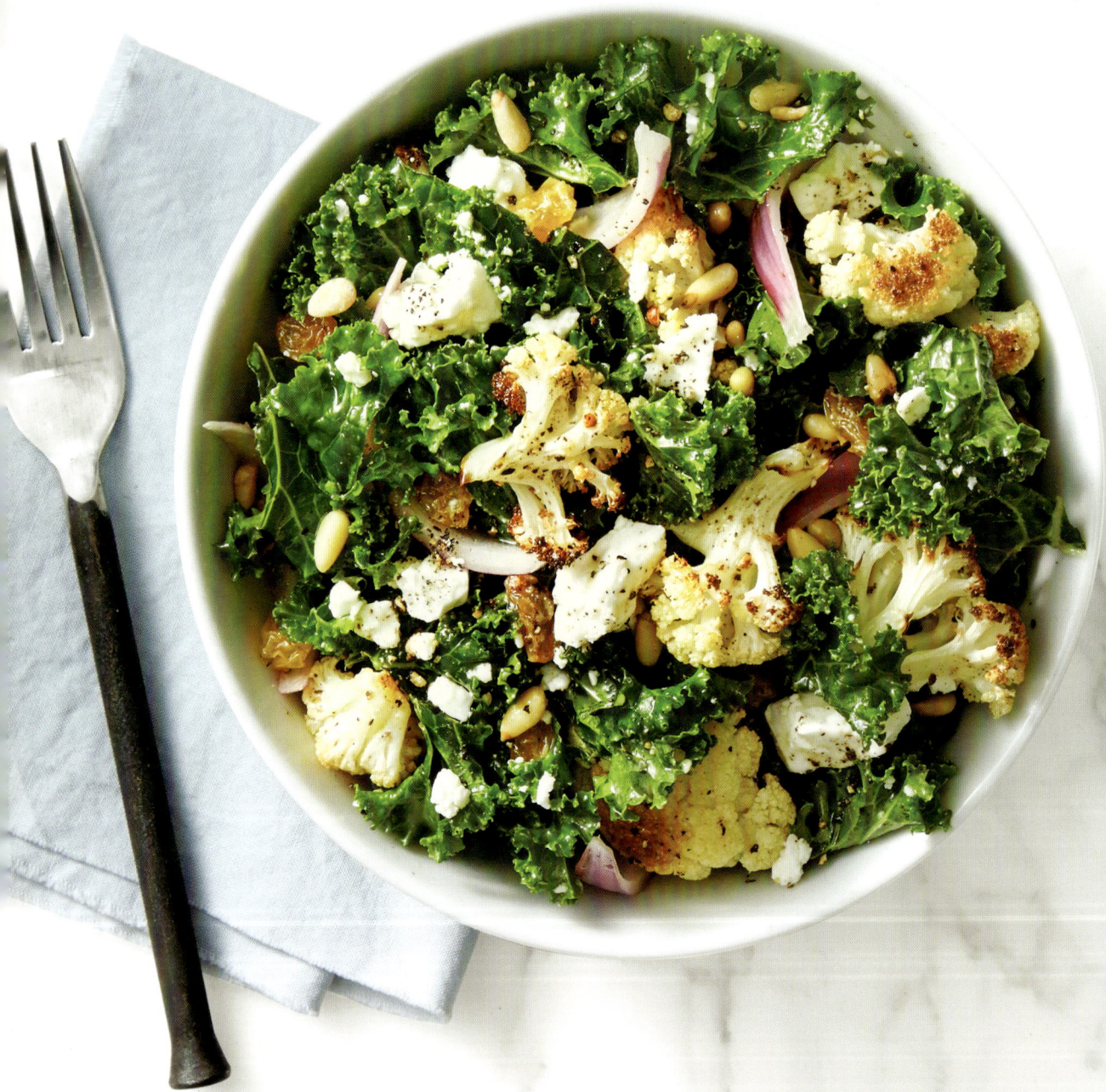

VEGETARIAN   HIGH FIBER

Kale and Roasted Cauliflower Salad

ACTIVE **25 MIN**. // TOTAL **25 MIN**. // SERVES **2**

Roasted cauliflower and fresh kale come together in this low-calorie salad recipe designed to keep your heart healthy and your belly full.

½	**lb cauliflower florets**
2½	**Tbsp olive oil, divided**
	Kosher salt and pepper
2	**Tbsp lemon juice**
	Kosher salt
¼	**small red onion, very thinly sliced**
½	**bunch kale, ribs removed, leaves chopped**
2½	**Tbsp crumbled feta cheese**
2½	**Tbsp golden raisins**
2½	**Tbsp toasted pine nuts**

1. Heat oven to 450°F. On a large rimmed baking sheet, toss cauliflower with 1 Tbsp oil and pinch each salt and pepper. Roast until golden brown and just tender, 15 to 20 min.

2. Meanwhile, in bowl, whisk together lemon juice, remaining 1½ Tbsp oil, and ¼ tsp salt. Stir in onion, then toss with kale to coat; let sit for 5 min.

3. Add cauliflower to kale along with onion, feta, raisins, and pine nuts and toss to combine.

PER SERVING
365 cal, 9 g pro, 27 g carb, 6 g fiber, 13 g sugars (0 g added sugars), 28 g fat (5 g sat fat), 475 mg sodium

LEFTOVER TIP
Store kale, cauliflower and remaining ingredients separately for up to 2 days. Toss together just before serving.

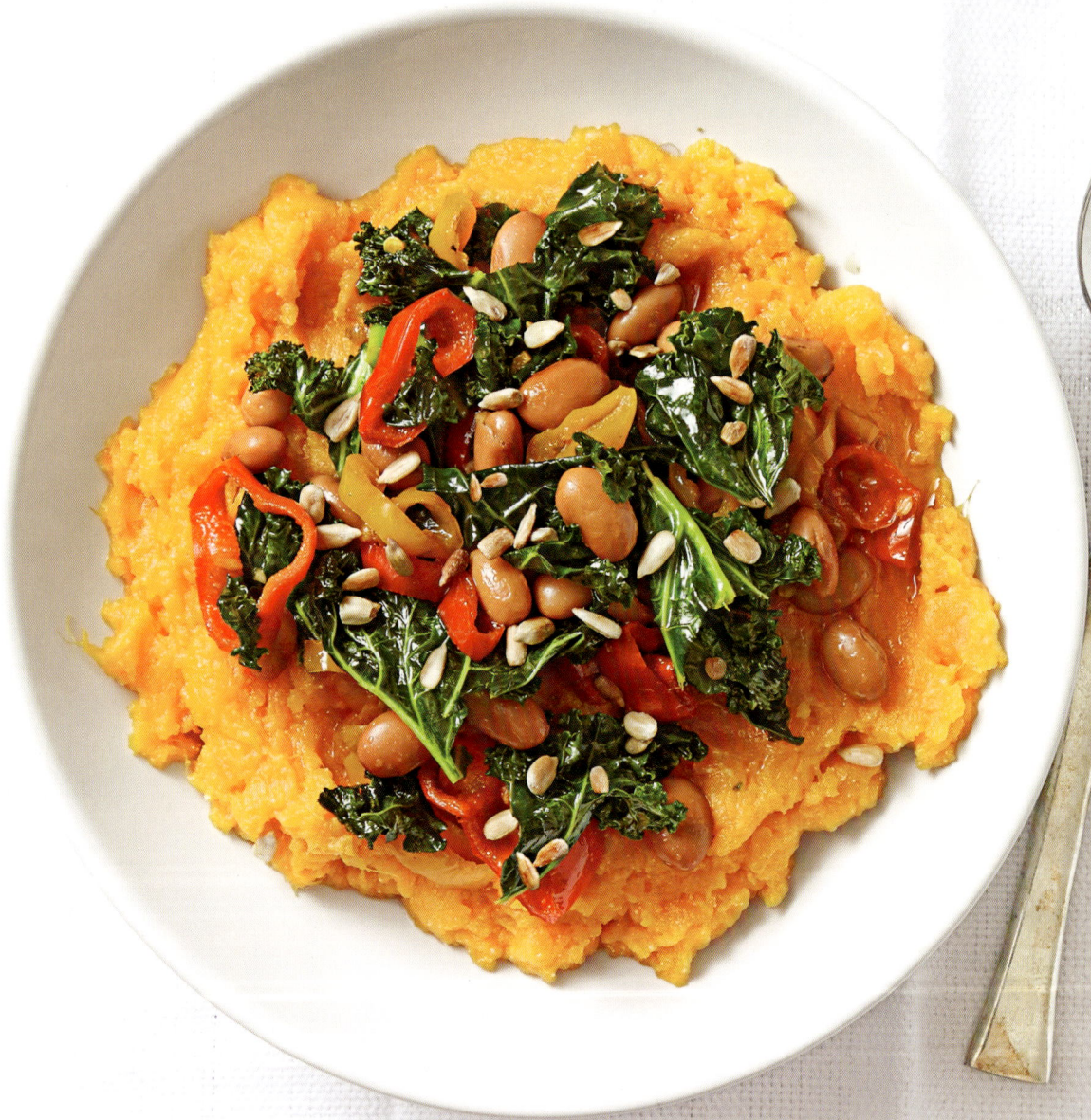

VEGETARIAN HIGH FIBER PROTEIN-PACKED

Veggie Medley on Sweet Potato

ACTIVE **25 MIN**. // TOTAL **25 MIN**. // SERVES **4**

Carbs aren't necessarily bad. In the case of sweet potatoes, they contain complex carbohydrates that take longer for your body to digest, which leads to more sustained energy. Sweet potatoes are also packed with potassium, which makes this dish a great lunch option to give your body the pre-workout fuel needed for a tough afternoon sweat session.

4	large sweet potatoes, peeled and cut into 1-in. chunks
	Kosher salt
3	oz Greek yogurt
2	Tbsp butter
1	Tbsp olive oil
3	cloves garlic, chopped
12	oz mini sweet peppers, sliced
1	bunch kale, chopped
	Black pepper
1	15-oz can pinto beans, drained
1	Tbsp lemon juice
1	Tbsp Worcestershire sauce
¼	cup sunflower seeds

1. Place sweet potatoes in a large pot and cover with water. Partially cover and bring to a boil. Add 1 tsp salt, reduce heat and simmer until tender, about 10 min. Drain and mash with yogurt and butter.

2. Meanwhile, heat oil and garlic in large skillet on medium until sizzling. Add peppers and sauté for 3 min. Add kale, season with ½ tsp each salt and pepper and cook, covered, tossing occasionally, until wilted and just tender, 5 to 6 min.

3. Toss with beans, lemon juice and Worcestershire and cook, tossing, until beans are heated through. Serve over mash and top with sunflower seeds.

PER SERVING
470 cal, 18 g pro, 66 g carb, 9 g fiber, 16 g sugars (0 g added sugars), 17 g fat (5 g sat fat), 760 mg sodium

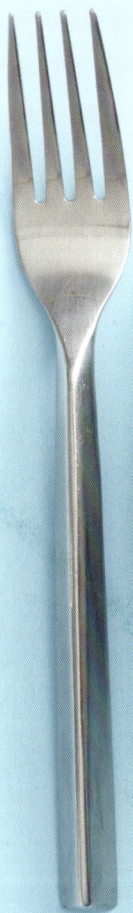
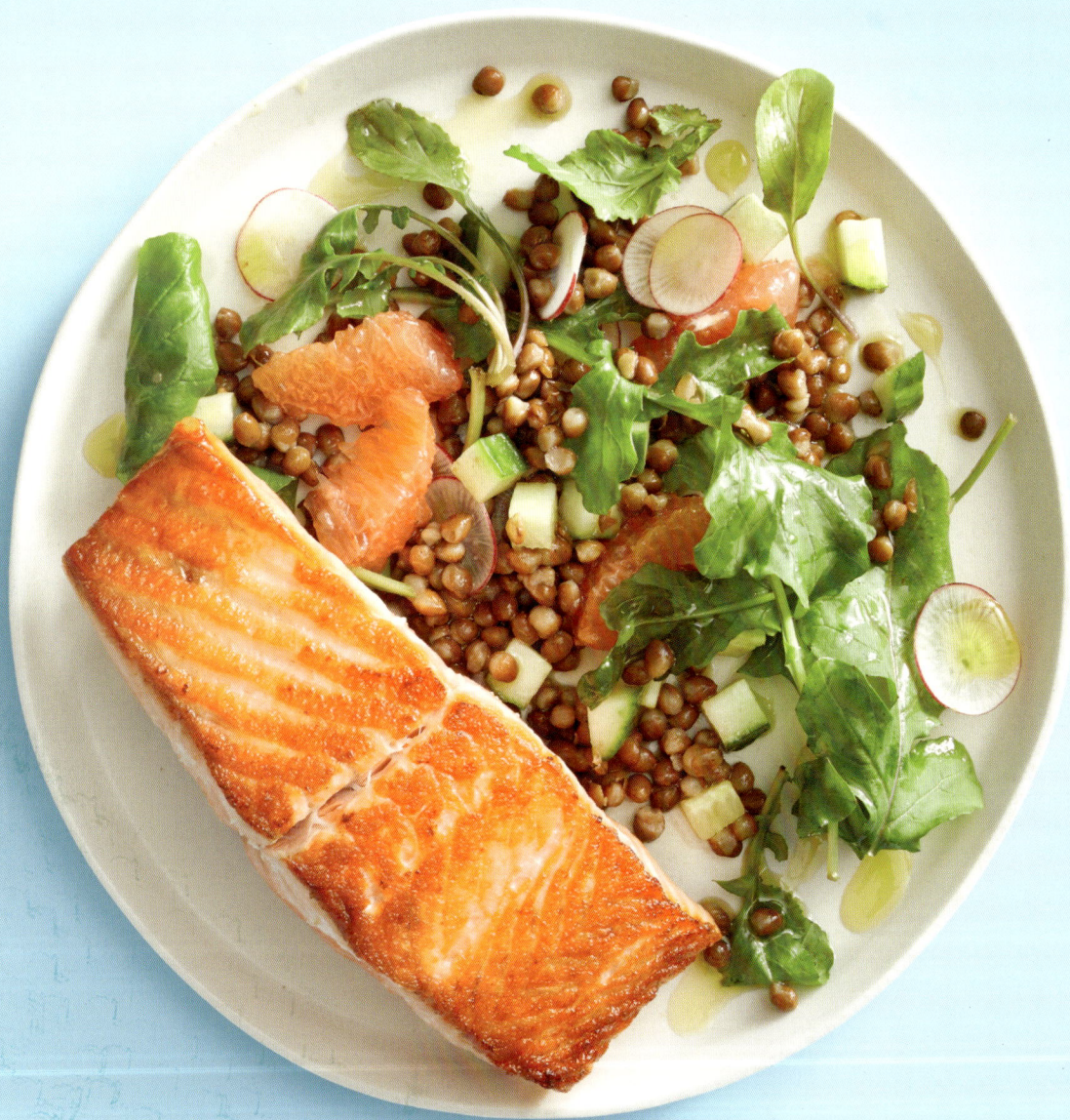

HIGH FIBER   PROTEIN-PACKED

Salmon with Grapefruit and Lentil Salad

ACTIVE **10 MIN**. // TOTAL **15 MIN**. // SERVES **1**

This hearty meal doesn't just boast protein-packed lentils and heart-healthy salmon, it also only takes 15 minutes to cook.

½	**Tbsp olive oil**
1	**5-oz piece skinless salmon fillet**
	Kosher salt and pepper
½	**Tbsp red wine vinegar**
⅓	**cup canned lentils, rinsed**
1	**small Persian cucumber, cut into pieces**
½	**small pink grapefruit, peel and pith removed, cut into pieces**
1	**radish, thinly sliced**
1½	**cups arugula**

1. Heat ½ Tbsp oil in small nonstick skillet on medium. Season salmon with pinch each salt and pepper and cook until golden brown, about 7 min. Turn salmon over and continue cooking until just opaque throughout, about 2 min. more.

2. Meanwhile, in a large bowl, whisk together vinegar and remaining ½ Tbsp oil. Add lentils and toss to coat, then add cucumber, grapefruit, and radishes and toss. Fold in arugula and serve with salmon.

PER SERVING
345 cal, 36 g pro, 23 g carb, 8 g fiber, 10 g sugars (0 g added sugars), 12.5 g fat (2 g sat fat), 260 mg sodium

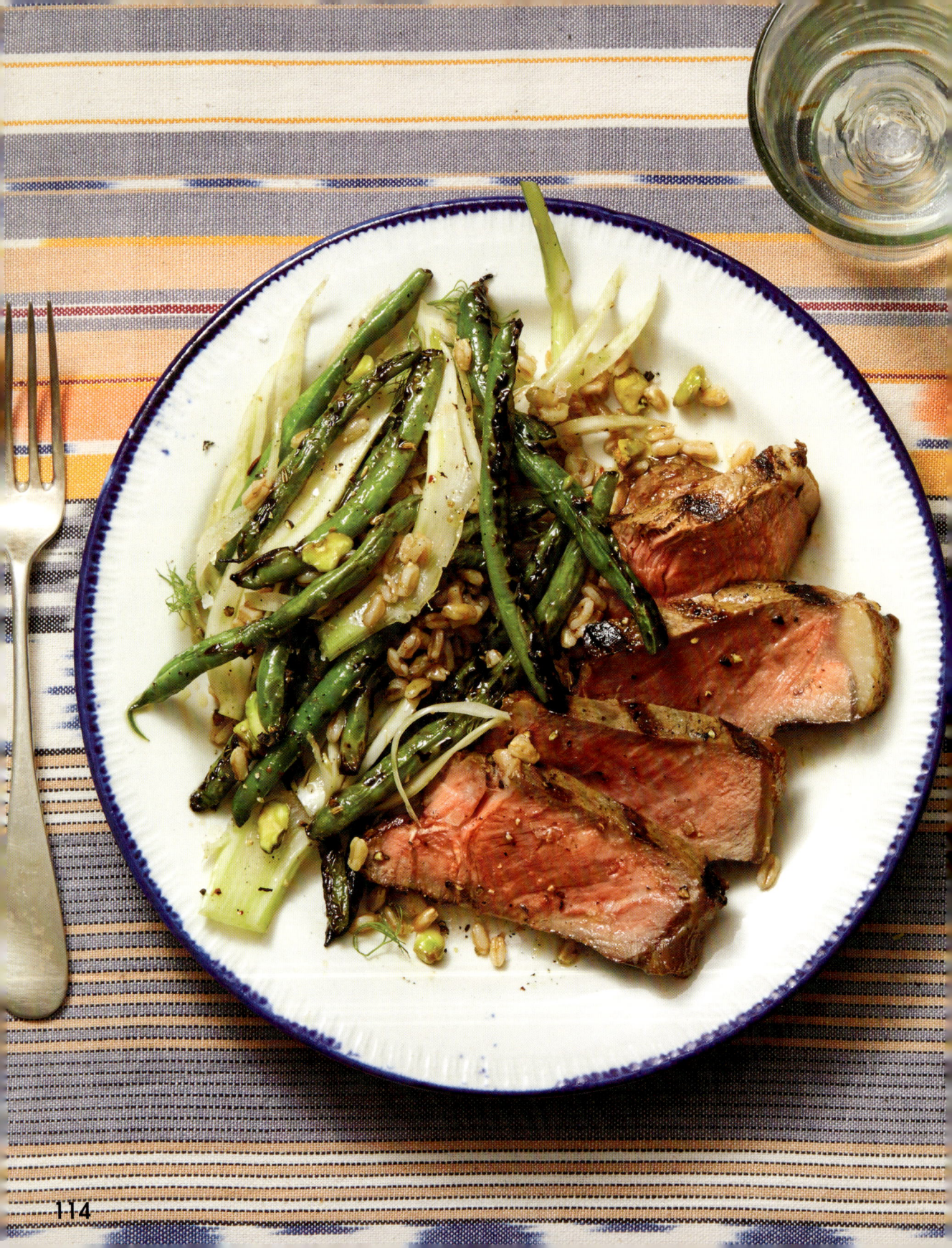

HIGH FIBER   PROTEIN-PACKED

Steak with Grilled Green Beans, Fennel & Farro

ACTIVE **25 MIN**. // TOTAL **25 MIN**. // SERVES **2**

Farro—a staple for ancient Egyptians and modern-day Italians alike—has everything you need: nearly twice the protein and fiber of brown rice, along with calcium and iron. Fire up the grill to char green beans and steak to go with it and you've got yourself the ultimate post-workout summer dinner.

¼ **cup quick-cooking farro**

¾ **lb strip or sirloin steak**

   Kosher salt and pepper

½ **lb green or wax beans, or a combination, trimmed**

1 **Tbsp plus 2 tsp olive oil, divided**

½ **Tbsp fennel seeds**

   Pinch red pepper flakes

1 **Tbsp white wine vinegar**

½ **tsp honey**

2 **Tbsp toasted pistachios, chopped**

½ **small bulb fennel, very thinly shaved**

   Fennel fronds, for serving

1. Cook farro per package directions. Drain, transfer to large bowl, and let cool to room temperature.

2. Heat grill to medium-high. Season steak with ½ tsp each salt and pepper and grill to desired doneness, 4 to 8 min. per side for medium-rare (depending on thickness). Transfer to a cutting board and let rest.

3. Meanwhile, in second bowl, toss green and wax beans with 2 tsp oil and ¼ tsp salt. Grill beans, turning occasionally, until just tender, 4 to 6 min. Transfer to bowl with farro.

4. In small skillet on medium, toast fennel seeds and pepper flakes until fragrant, about 2 min. Let cool, then pulse in spice grinder (or crush with side of heavy skillet) until mostly cracked.

5. While spices are cooling, in small bowl, whisk together vinegar, honey, remaining Tbsp oil and ¼ tsp salt. Stir in fennel seed mixture and pistachios. Toss farro and beans with dressing and fold in fennel. Slice steak and serve with farro salad, topped with fennel fronds if desired.

PER SERVING
550 cal, 43 g pro,
31 g carb, 7 g fiber,
7 g sugars
(1 g added sugars),
29 g fat
(7.5 g sat fat),
1,080 mg sodium

HIGH FIBER   PROTEIN-PACKED

Greek Chicken Grain Bowl

ACTIVE **15 MIN**. // TOTAL **15 MIN**. // SERVES **2**

LEFTOVER TIP
Refrigerate the second portion for up to 2 days. Spoon into an airtight container with each of the components side by side instead of top, then dollop with yogurt and feta just before serving or packing to go.

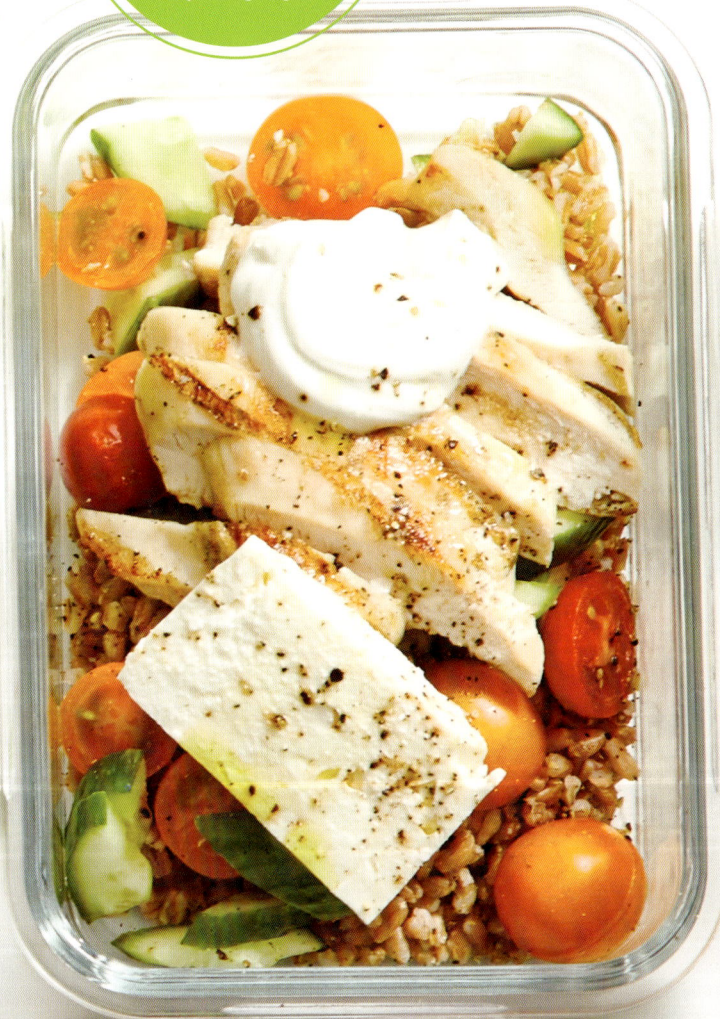

Put together this healthy, delicious meal in advance, then just grab and go when you need to head out the door.

- ½   cup farro
- 2   6-oz boneless skinless chicken breasts
- 2   Tbsp olive oil, divided
      Kosher salt and pepper
- 1   lemon, halved
- 1   cup cherry or grape tomatoes, halved
- 2   small Persian cucumbers, diced
      Plain Greek yogurt and feta cheese, for serving

1. Heat grill to medium-high. Cook farro per package directions.

2. Meanwhile, brush chicken with ½ Tbsp oil and season with ¼ tsp each salt and pepper. Grill until just cooked through, 5 to 6 min. per side. Squeeze juice from half of lemon over the top, then transfer to a cutting board and let rest 5 min. before slicing.

3. Toss tomatoes and cucumbers with remaining 1½ Tbsp oil, 1 Tbsp lemon juice and a pinch each of salt and pepper.

4. Divide farro among 2 bowls, and top with tomato mixture and chicken. Dollop with yogurt and add a small piece of feta cheese, if desired.

PER SERVING 475 cal, 11 g pro, 66 g carb, 9 g fiber, 37 g sugars (12 g added sugars), 20 g fat (3 g sat fat), 290 mg sodium

HIGH FIBER   PROTEIN-PACKED

Hearty Breakfast Egg Sandwich

ACTIVE **15 MIN.** // TOTAL **15 MIN.** // SERVES **1**

Breakfast sandwiches are a nice break from the bagel-and-cream-cheese routine. This one combines creamy mashed avocado, fresh tomatoes, filling eggs, and savory Cheddar in a whole-wheat English muffin for the ultimate energy boost to start your day right.

1   **whole egg**

1   **egg white**

1   **whole-wheat English muffin, toasted**

¼   **cup Hass avocado, mashed**

1   **slice reduced-fat Cheddar cheese**

2   **tomato slices**

1. In a skillet coated with cooking spray, scramble egg with egg white.

2. Spread English muffin with avocado, and top with scrambled eggs, cheese, and tomato.

PER SERVING
355 cal, 23 g pro,
32 g carb, 8 g fiber,
7 g sugars
(5 g added sugars),
16.5 g fat
(5 g sat fat),
495 mg sodium

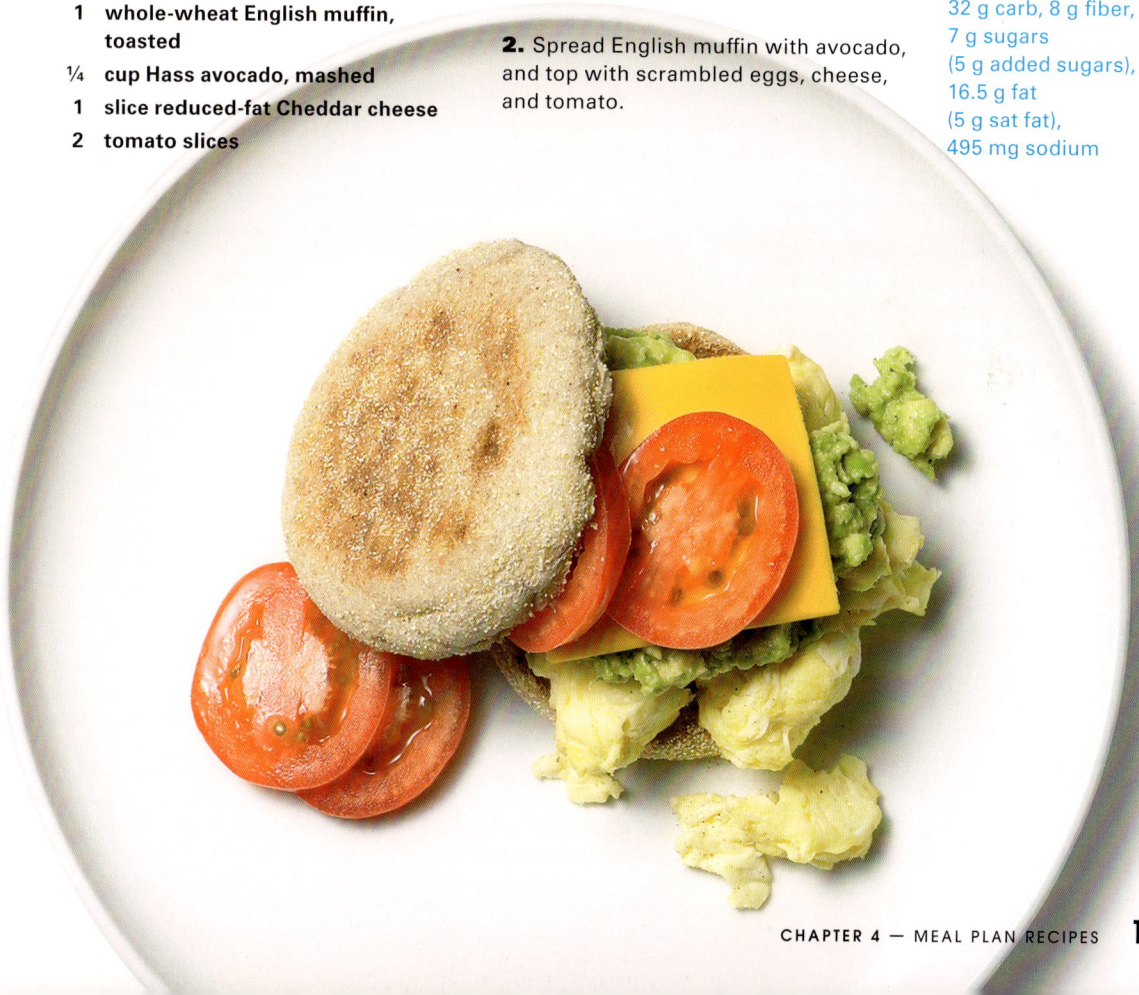

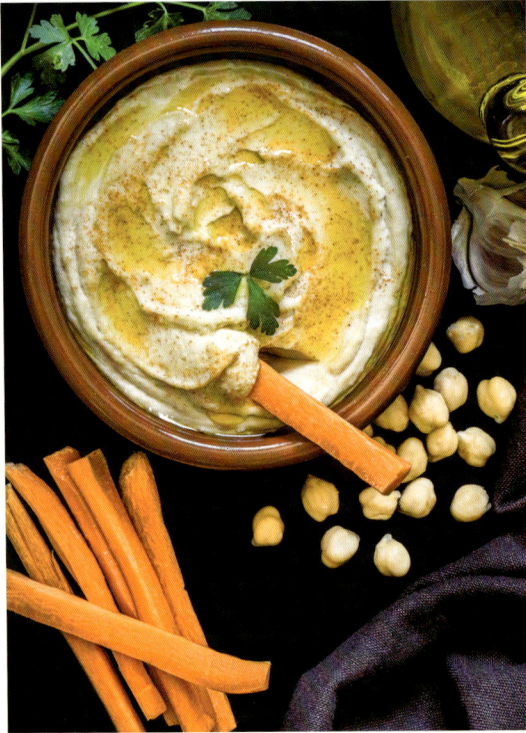

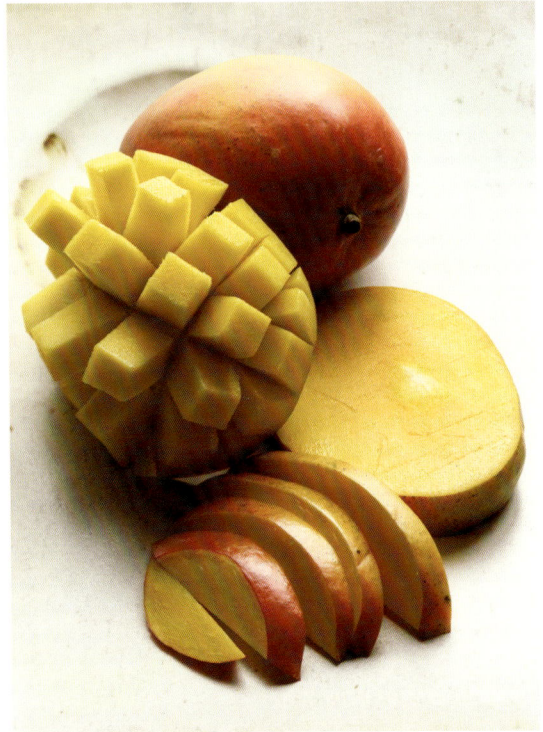

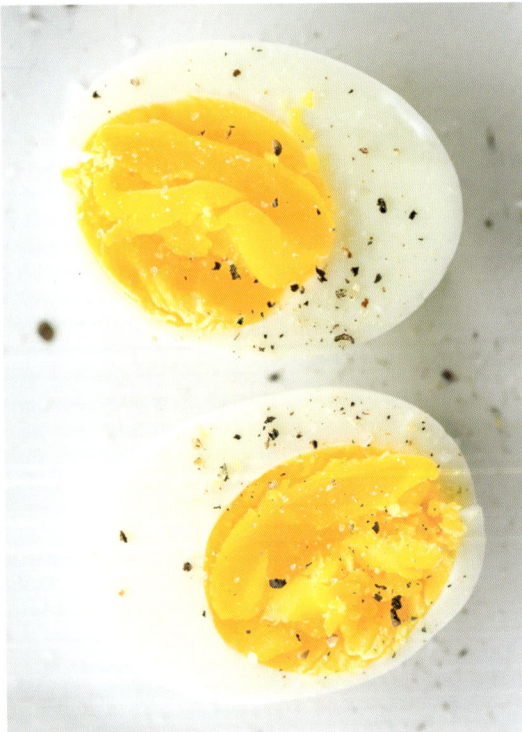

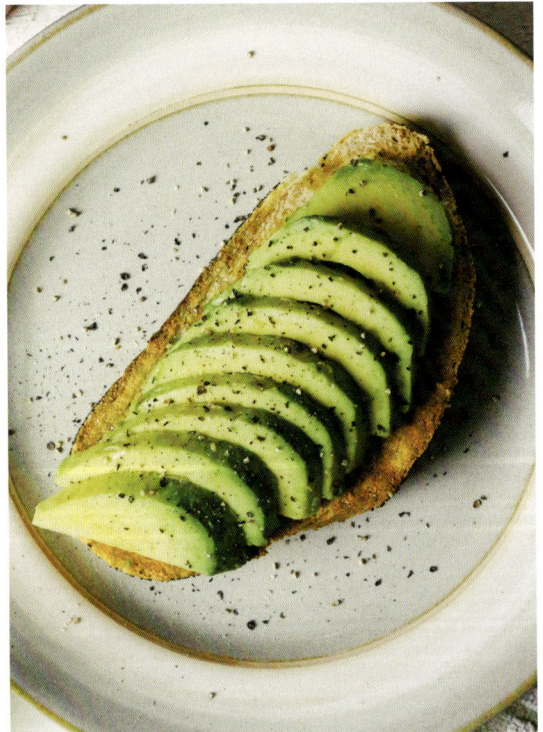

Snacks & Extras

Healthy snacks are a big part of feeling great on this plan, and we've included one each day. You can use them whenever you like, but most people will need a snack in the late morning or late afternoon. We've designed them to have a balanced combination of carbohydrates, protein, and healthy fat.

Almonds + Banana

1 oz almonds (23 nuts) + medium banana =
PER SERVING 270 cal, 7 g pro, 33 g carb, 7 g fiber, 16 g sugars (0 g added sugars), 14.5 g fat (1 g sat fat), 0 mg sodium

Hummus + Carrots

¼ cup hummus + ⅔ cup baby carrots =
PER SERVING 170 cal, 5 g pro, 15 g carb, 4 g fiber, 4 g sugars (0 g added sugars), 10 g fat, 2 g sat fat), 325 mg sodium

Banana + Peanut Butter

Banana + 1 peanut butter squeeze pack =
PER SERVING 375 cal, 10 g pro, 34 g carb, 5 g fiber, 18 g sugars (0 g added sugars), 23.5 g fat (5 g sat fat), 230 mg sodium

Melon + Pistachios

2 cups cubed melon (any variety) + ½ oz pistachios =
PER SERVING 200 cal, 5 g pro, 33 g carb, 4 g fiber, 27 g sugars (0 g added sugars), 7 g fat (1 g sat fat), 55 mg sodium

Apple + Almonds

Apple + 12 almonds =
PER SERVING 180 cal, 4 g pro, 28 g carb, 6 g fiber, 20 g sugars (0 g added sugars), 7.5 g fat (0.5 g sat fat), 0 mg sodium

Grapes + Cashews

1 cup grapes + 1 oz cashews (20 whole cashews) =
PER SERVING 265 cal, 5 g pro, 37 g carb, 2 g fiber, 25 g sugars (0 g added sugars), 13.5 g fat (2.5 g sat fat), 5 mg sodium

Apple + Cashews

Apple + 1 oz cashews (20 whole cashews) =
PER SERVING 260 cal, 5 g pro, 34 g carb, 5 g fiber, 20 g sugars (0 g sugars), 13.5 g fat (2.5 g sat fat), 5 mg sodium

Yogurt + Walnuts

5.3-oz vanilla Greek whole milk yogurt + 7 walnuts =
PER SERVING 240 cal, 15 g pro, 16 g carb, 1 g fiber, 12 g sugars (8 g added sugars), 14 g fat (3.5 g sat fat), 50 mg sodium

Mango + Cashew Butter

1 cup fresh mango + 1 Tbsp cashew butter =
PER SERVING 195 cal, 3 g pro, 30 g carb, 4 g fiber, 23 g sugars (0 g added sugars), 30.5 g fat (2 g sat fat), 45 mg sodium

Orange + Cheese

Navel orange + cheese stick =
PER SERVING 140 cal, 6 g pro, 19 g carb, 3 g fiber, 13 g sugars (0 g added sugars), 6.5 g fat (4 g sat fat), 170 mg sodium

Hard-Boiled Egg

1 egg =
PER SERVING 80 cal, 6 g pro, 0 g carb, 0 g fiber, 0 g sugar (0 g added sugars), 5.5 g fat (1.5 g sat fat), 60 mg sodium

Almond Butter Toast

1 slice of whole-grain bread (about 100 calories) + 1 Tbsp almond butter =
PER SERVING 210 cal, 8 g pro, 23 g carb, 5 g fiber, 5 g sugars (3 g added sugars), 10 g fat (1 g sat fat), 150 mg sodium

Avocado Toast

1 slice of whole-grain bread (about 100 calories) + ⅓ avocado =
PER SERVING 215 cal, 6 g pro, 26 g carb, 7 g fiber, 4 g sugars (3 g added sugars), 10.5 g fat (1.5 g sat fat), 155 mg sodium

CHAPTER 5

Bonus Smoothie Recipes

Feel free to replace any of the smoothies in the 28-day plan with one of these recipes, or use them to continue your smoothie-a-day routine!

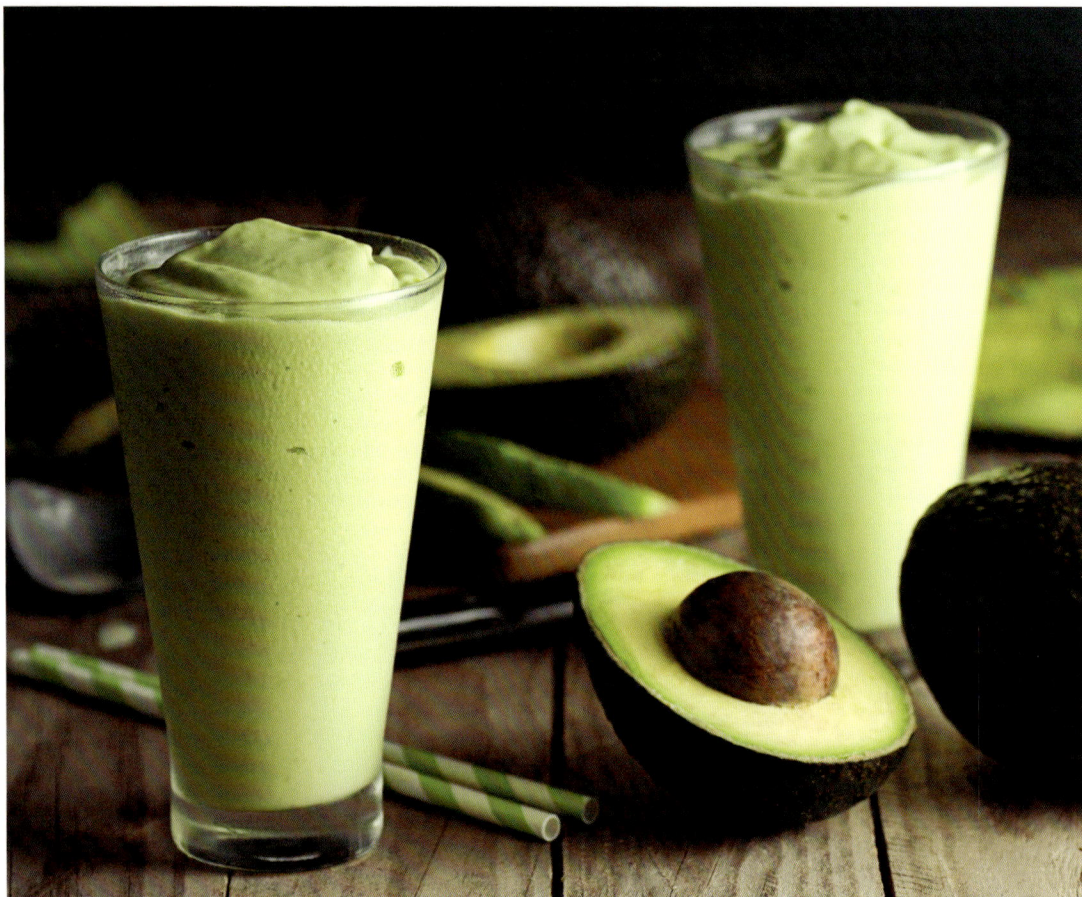

Green Dream Smoothie

TOTAL **5 MIN**. // SERVES **1**

You might not know this, but avocado is actually loaded with fiber. Half an avocado boasts about 7 grams of fiber, making it an excellent addition to any smoothie. We love starting our day with this creamy green one.

½ **cup unsweetened refrigerated vanilla almond milk**

¼ **cup whole milk vanilla yogurt**

¼ **tsp ground cinnamon**

⅓ **ripe avocado**

½ **large banana**

1 **cup baby spinach**

¼ **cup ice**

In a blender, combine all ingredients and puree until smooth.

PER SERVING
260 cal, 7 g pro,
32 g carb, 8 g fiber,
17 g sugars (4 g
added sugars),
13 g fat
(2.5 g sat fat),
165 mg sodium

Coconut-Cherry Blast

TOTAL **10 MIN.** // SERVES **1**

Cherries contain 3 grams of fiber and 342 milligrams of potassium per cup, which is about the same as a small banana. This garnet fruit also contains anthocyanins, which give cherries their deep red color and contributes the anti-inflammatory benefits.

- ½ **cup unsweetened coconut milk, refrigerated**
- 1 **Tbsp creamy almond butter**
- ½ **cup fresh or frozen pitted sweet cherries**
- ¼ **cup ice**

In a blender, combine all ingredients and puree until smooth.

PER SERVING 170 cal, 4 g pro, 15 g carb, 3 g fiber, 10 g sugars (0 g added sugars), 11.5 g fat (3 g sat fat), 10 mg sodium

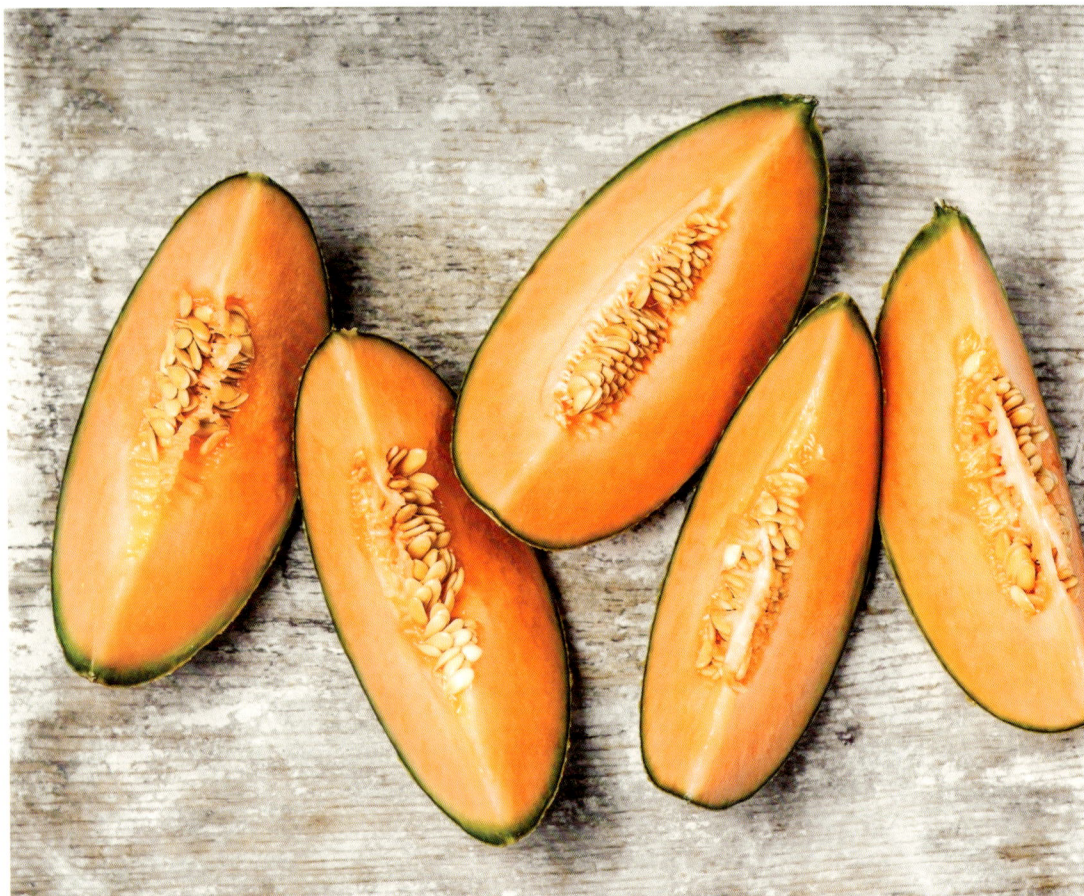

Mango-Melon Smoothie

VEGAN
HIGH FIBER

TOTAL **5 MIN**. // SERVES **1**

We love the tropical flavors in this pretty smoothie. And we also like that the beta-carotene in the cantaloupe and mango help provide our skin with natural SPF! Sip this before a day at the beach for extra protection in addition to your usual sunscreen.

½ **cup unsweetened refrigerated coconut milk**
1 **Tbsp fresh lime juice**
1 **Tbsp coconut butter**
1 **cup cubed cantaloupe**
1 **cup cubed fresh or frozen mango**
1 **banana**
   Coconut chips, for garnish, optional

In a blender, combine all ingredients and puree until smooth.

PER SERVING
380 cal, 6 g pro, 70 g carb, 10 g fiber, 50 g sugars (0 g added sugars), 13 g fat (11 g sat fat), 40 mg sodium

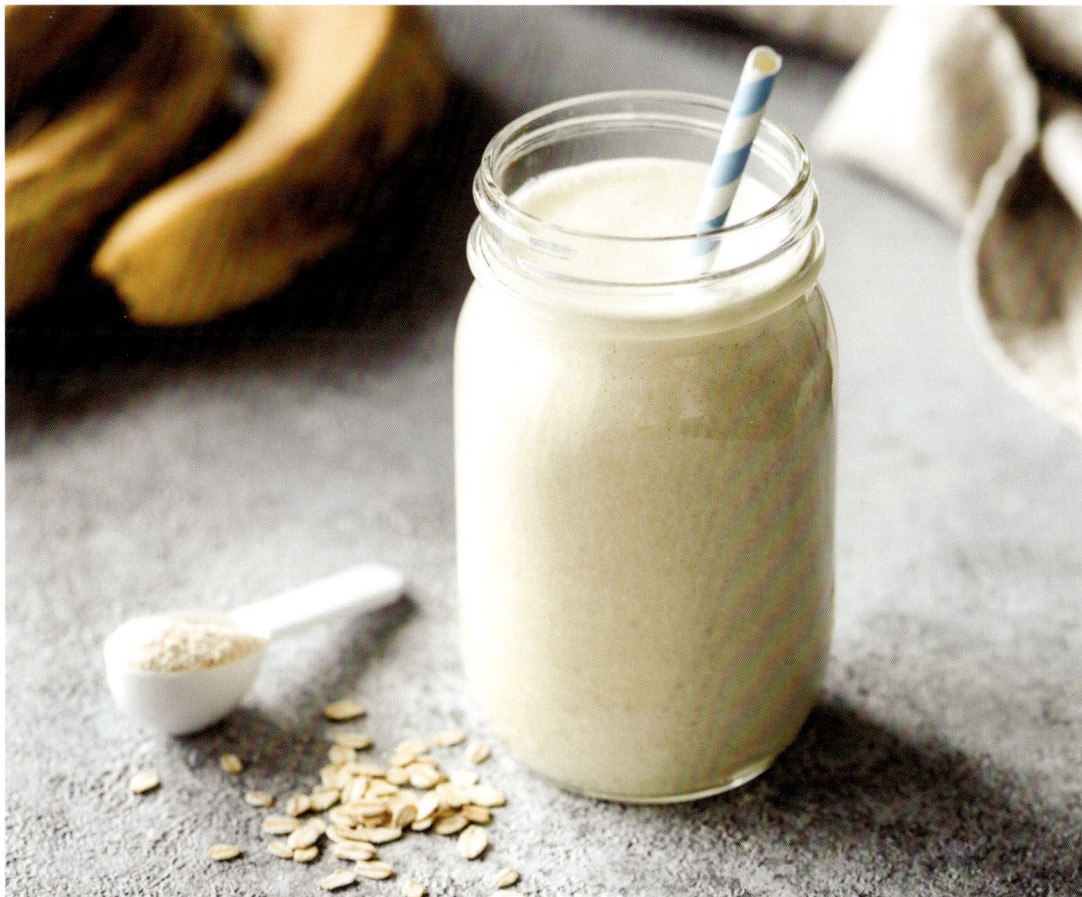

Oaty Nut Smoothie

VEGAN
PROTEIN-PACKED
HIGH FIBER

TOTAL **5 MIN**. // SERVES **1**

Looking for a filling and power-packed post-workout smoothie? Coming right up! With satisfying oats, natural sweetness from dates and banana, and plenty of protein to fuel your muscles, this hearty smoothie will keep you going all morning.

1   **cup unsweetened oat milk**
1   **pitted date**
1   **Tbsp creamy peanut butter**
1   **scoop vanilla protein powder (preferably plant-based)**
¼   **cup rolled oats**
1   **banana**
¼   **cup ice**

In a blender, combine all ingredients and puree until smooth.

PER SERVING
470 cal, 39 g pro,
56 g carb, 7 g fiber,
22 g sugars
(1 g added sugars),
13.5 g fat
(2 g sat fat),
330 mg sodium

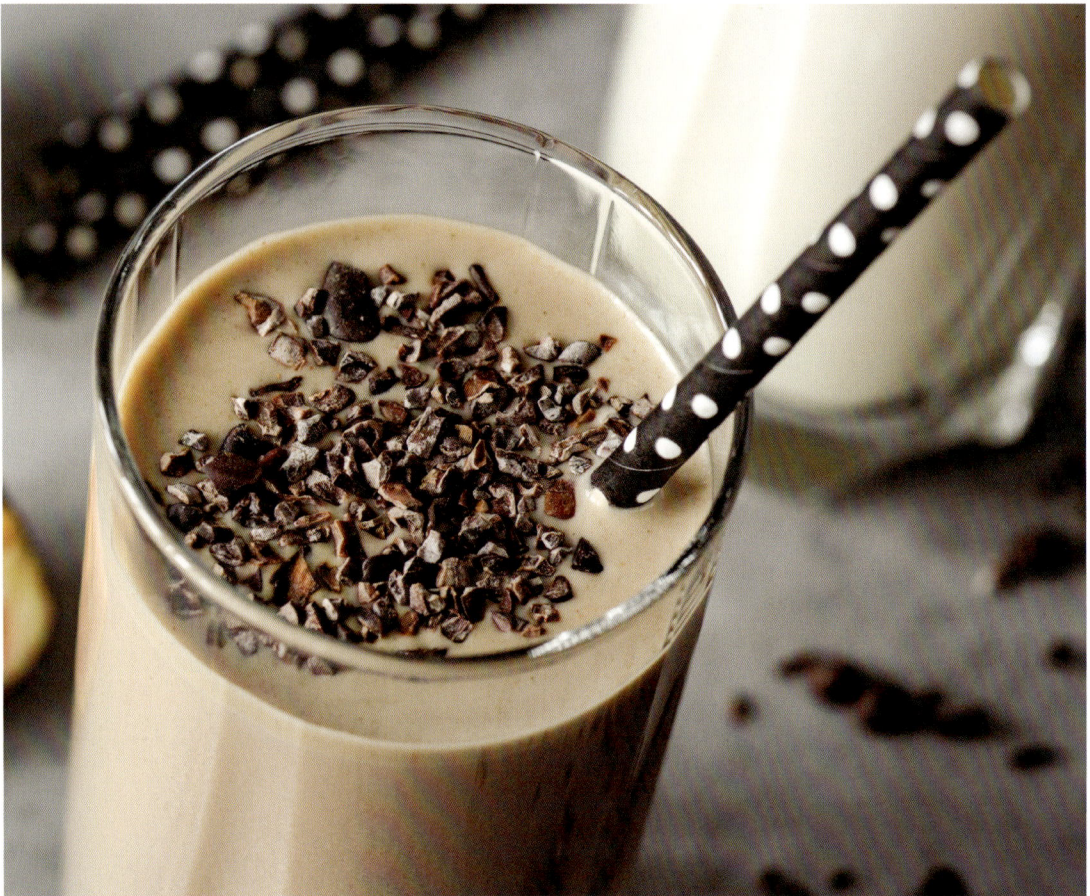

Cacao Blast Smoothie

VEGAN
HIGH FIBER

TOTAL **5 MIN**. // SERVES **1**

Some days require an extra caffeine boost to get them off the ground. This smoothie does just that with a combination of cold brew, cacao nibs, and almond butter. It's an excellent pre-workout smoothie and is also great for getting you going on your morning commute.

½	**cup cold brew (not from concentrate)**
½	**cup chocolate oat milk**
2	**tsp cacao nibs**
1	**Tbsp almond butter**
½	**banana**
¼	**cup ice**

In a blender, combine all ingredients and puree until smooth.

PER SERVING
280 cal, 7 g pro, 33 g carb, 8 g fiber, 16 g sugars (8 g added sugars), 13.5 g fat (2 g sat fat), 80 mg sodium

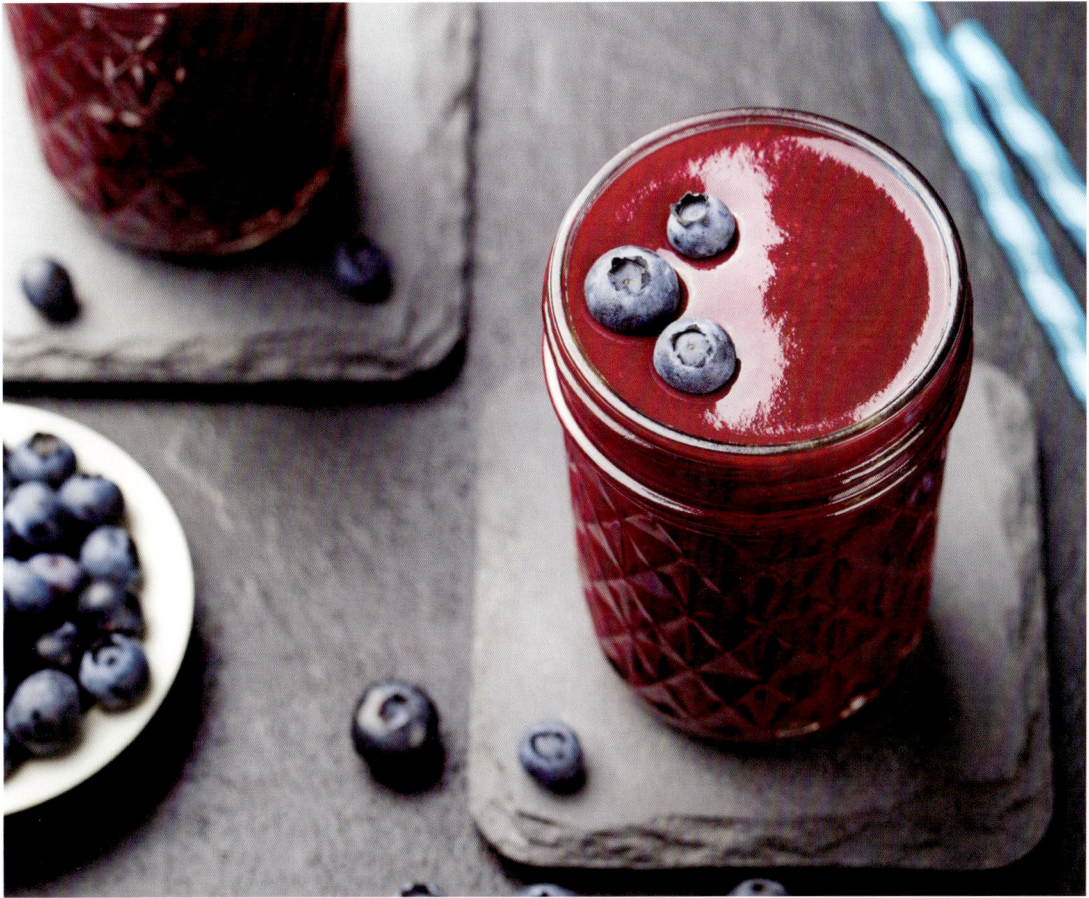

Berry Palooza Smoothie

PROTEIN-PACKED

TOTAL **5 MIN.** // SERVES **1**

Looking for a satisfying smoothie with major berry flavor? We've got you covered with this rich-tasting, creamy smoothie. It's loaded with the antioxidant power of three types of berries. The added protein makes it perfect for a post-workout pick-me-up.

½ **cup vanilla whole milk yogurt**

½ **scoop vanilla protein powder**

1 **3.5-oz frozen acai pack**

¼ **cup strawberries, fresh or frozen**

¼ **cup blueberries, fresh or frozen**

In a blender, combine all ingredients and puree until smooth.

PER SERVING
290 cal, 22 g pro, 30 g carb, 4 g fiber, 23 g sugars (8 g added sugars), 9 g fat (3.5 g sat fat), 170 mg sodium

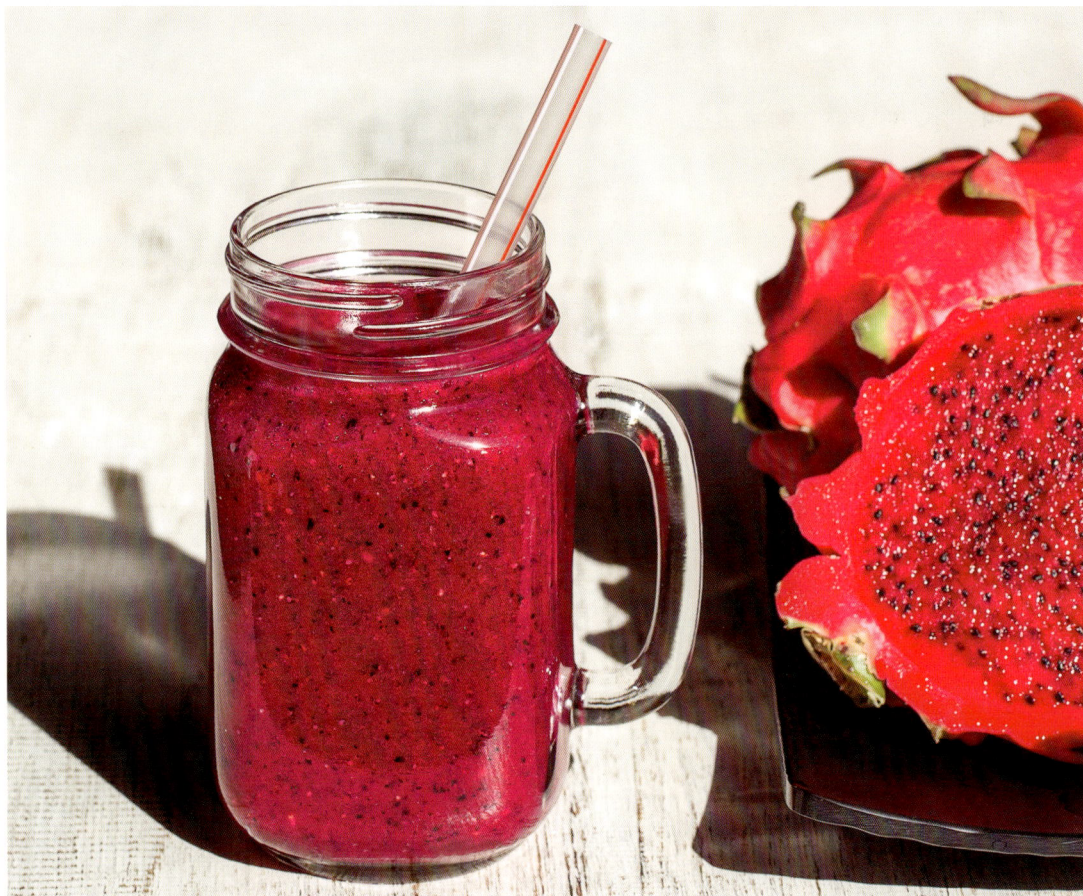

Dragon Fire Smoothie

VEGAN
HIGH FIBER

TOTAL **5 MIN.** // SERVES **1**

Want a metabolism boost? Blend up this fuchsia-colored drink and fire up your day. The pomegranate juice and the dragon fruit deliver serious antioxidants, while the cayenne pepper gives you a temporary metabolism boost—pow!

½ **cup pomegranate juice**

⅛ **tsp cayenne pepper**

1 **banana**

1 **packet frozen dragon fruit, defrosted (½ cup)**

½ **cup fresh or frozen cubed pineapple**

¼ **cup ice**

In a blender, combine all ingredients and puree until smooth.

PER SERVING
280 cal, 3 g pro,
68 g carb, 8 g fiber,
44 g sugars (0 g
added sugars),
1 g fat (0 g sat fat),
4 mg sodium

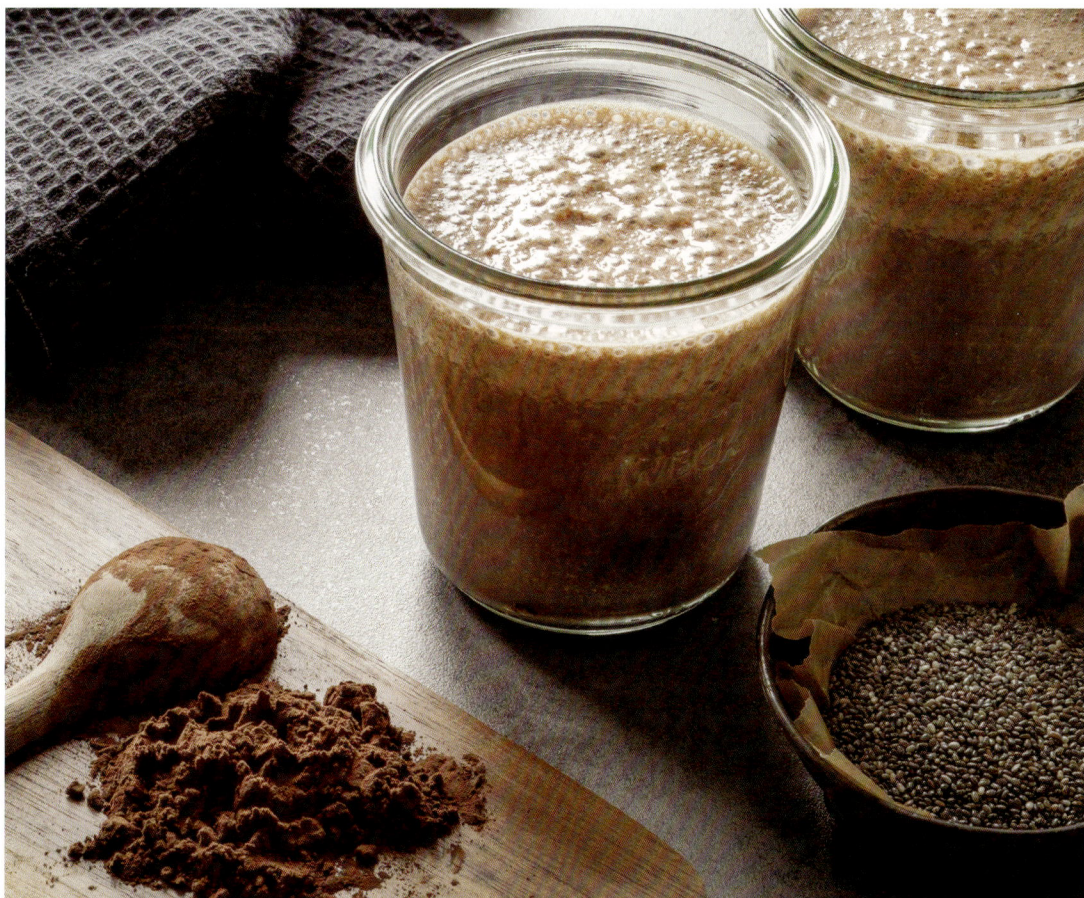

Chia-Chocolate-Cherry Chaser

VEGAN
HIGH FIBER

TOTAL **10 MIN**. // SERVES **1**

Got a chocolate craving? Get ready to indulge that sweet tooth with this super delicious and satisfying smoothie. And that cocoa powder doesn't just add a ton of flavor, it's also fabulous for your heart and your skin. Bottoms up!

½ **cup unsweetened vanilla almond milk**

1 **banana**

½ **cup pitted cherries, fresh or frozen**

2 **tsp chia seeds**

2 **tsp unsweetened cocoa powder**

¼ **cup ice**

In a blender, combine all ingredients and puree until smooth.

PER SERVING
215 cal, 4 g pro, 45 g carb, 8 g fiber, 24 g sugars (0 added sugars), 4.5 g fat (0.5 g sat fat), 90 g sodium

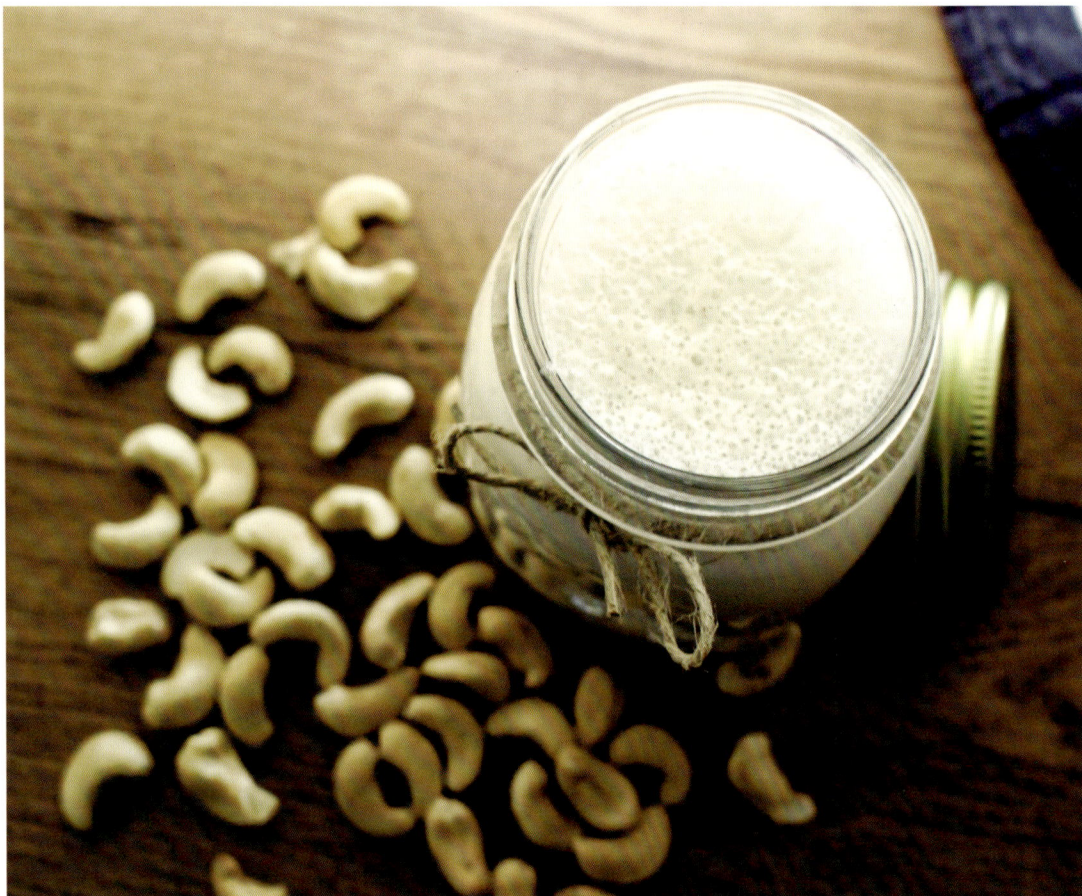

Cashew Dreams

VEGAN
HIGH FIBER

TOTAL **15 MIN**. // SERVES **1**

Milkshake lovers rejoice! This dairy-free, but oh-so-rich and creamy cashew smoothie is just as indulgent-tasting as a vanilla milkshake. And what's more, it serves up over 20 grams of muscle-building plant protein.

- 1 **cup unsweetened cashew milk**
- ¼ **cup raw cashews, soaked in water for 15 min. and drained**
- ¼ **tsp ground cinnamon**
- 1 **date**
- 1 **scoop vanilla plant protein powder**
- 1 **banana**
- ¼ **cup ice**

In a blender, combine all ingredients and puree until smooth.

PER SERVING
345 cal, 13 g pro, 46 g carb, 5 g fiber, 22 g sugars (1 g added sugars), 15 g fat (2.5 g sat fat), 265 mg sodium

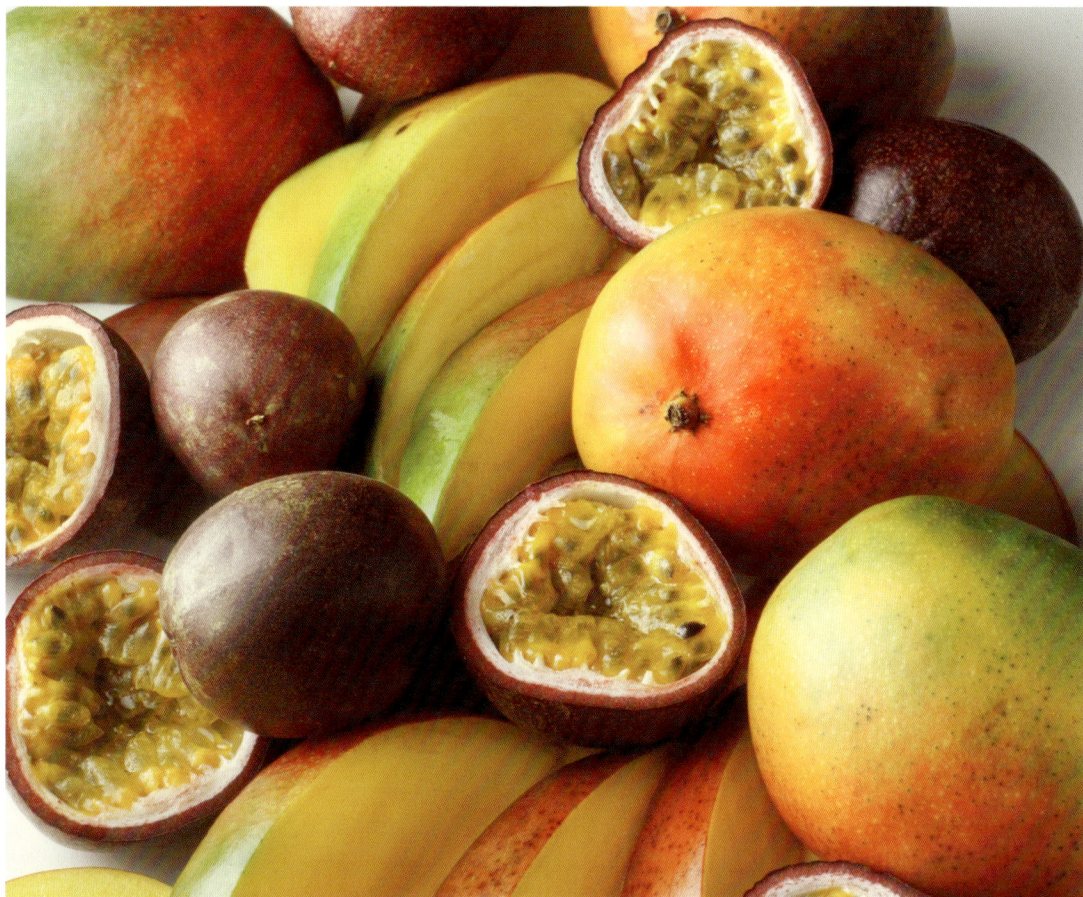

Mango-Passion Smoothie

HIGH FIBER

TOTAL **15 MIN.** // SERVES **1**

Tangy and tropical, with anti-inflammatory benefits from turmeric, this smoothie will leave you feeling energized and ready for whatever the day brings.

½ **cup unsweetened vanilla almond milk**

½ **tsp honey**

½ **cup fresh or frozen mango**

½ **cup fresh or frozen passion fruit**

¼ **cup raw cashews, soaked in water for 15 min. and drained**

¼ **tsp ground turmeric**

In a blender, combine all ingredients and puree until smooth.

PER SERVING
350 cal, 9 g pro, 52 g carb, 15 g fiber, 29 g sugars (3 g added sugars), 15 g fat (2.5 g sat fat), 125 mg sodium

VEGAN **HIGH FIBER**
PROTEIN-PACKED

Energizing Smoothie

TOTAL **5 MIN.** // SERVES **1**

Research has shown that bioactive compounds in ginger root, such as gingerols, can aid digestion and reduce inflammation. Jump-start your day with this refreshing smoothie that supports digestive health.

4	oz coconut water
1	banana
½-	in. piece of ginger root, peeled
1	cup baby kale
2	Tbsp vegan protein powder
2	Tbsp walnuts

In a blender, combine all ingredients and puree until smooth.

PER SERVING 295 cal, 17 g pro, 36 g carb, 5 g fiber, 20 g sugars (0 g added sugars), 11 g fat (1.5 g sat fat), 215 mg sodium

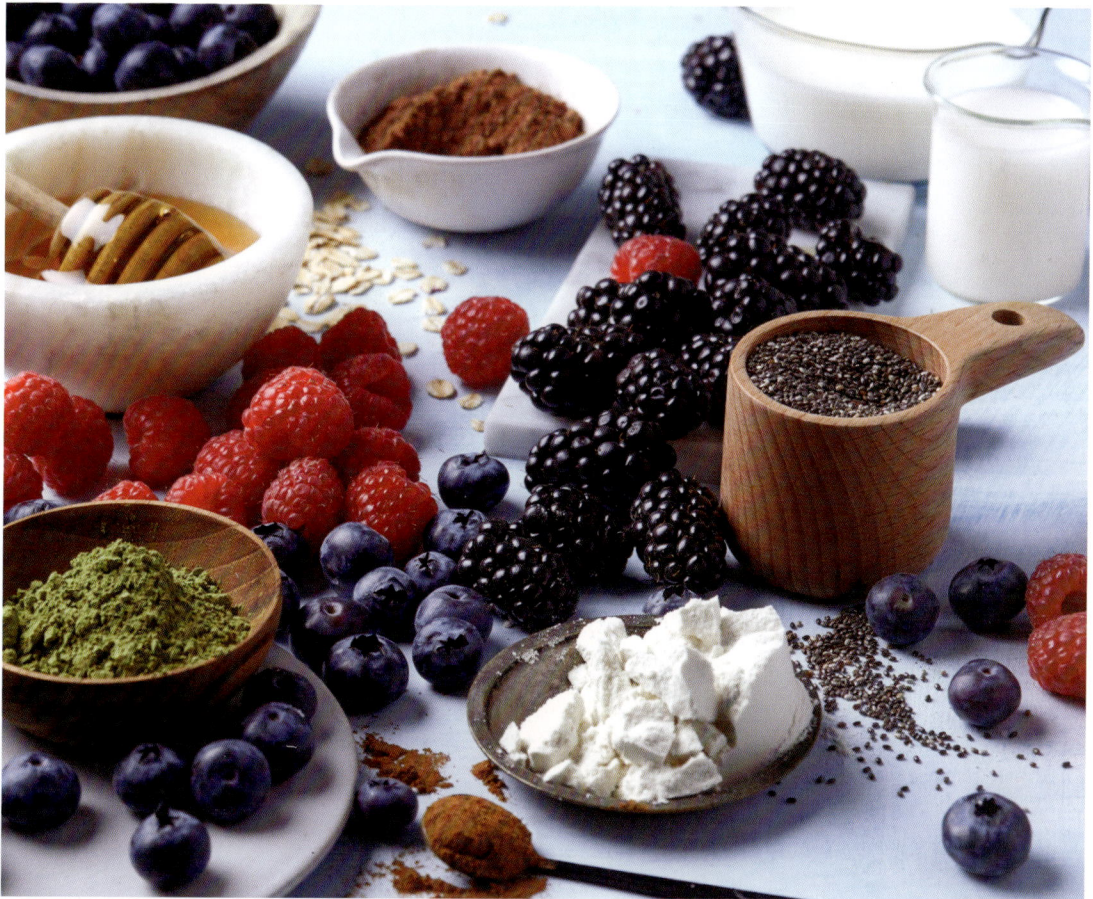

Mind Booster

TOTAL **5 MIN**. // SERVES **1**

Have a fresh start to your day and sip on this smoothie to support healthy brain function. The dark hues of those pretty jewel-toned berries come from high concentrations of anthocyanins, which research says may reduce inflammation and help keep your brain sharp.

1 cup unsweetened almond milk

⅓ cup vanilla whey protein powder

¼ tsp matcha powder

Dash of cinnamon

½ cup fresh or frozen blueberries

In a blender, combine all ingredients and puree until smooth.

PER SERVING
205 cal, 26 g pro, 16 g carb, 3 g fiber, 9 g sugars (2 g added sugars), 5 g fat (1.5 g sat fat), 285 mg sodium

Blueberry Banana-Nut Smoothie

TOTAL **5 MIN**. // SERVES **1**

Nut butters are a great substitute for peanut butter. A little nut butter can give you the protein boost your morning needs. And apart from being slightly sweeter, almond butter also has more calcium, vitamin E, and fill-you-up fiber than PB.

- 1 **cup unsweetened almond milk**
- 2 **Tbsp almond butter**
- 1 **banana, frozen**
- ½ **cup frozen blueberries**

In a blender, combine all ingredients and puree until smooth.

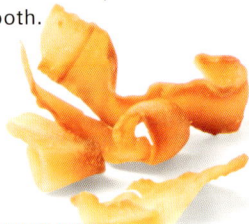

PER SERVING 380 cal, 9 g pro, 44 g carb, 9 g fiber, 22 g sugars (0 g added sugars), 21.5 g fat (1.5 g sat fat), 185 mg sodium

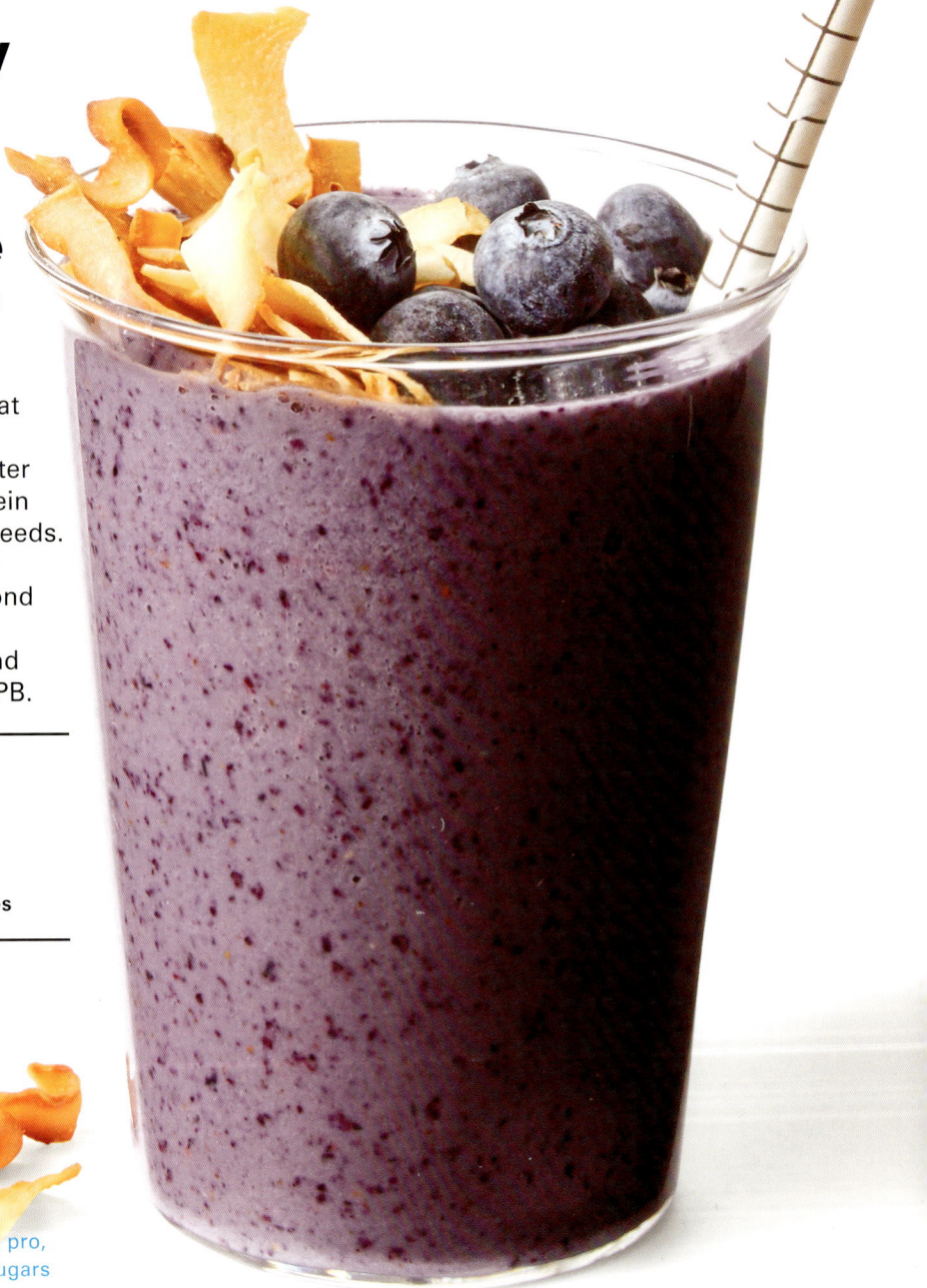

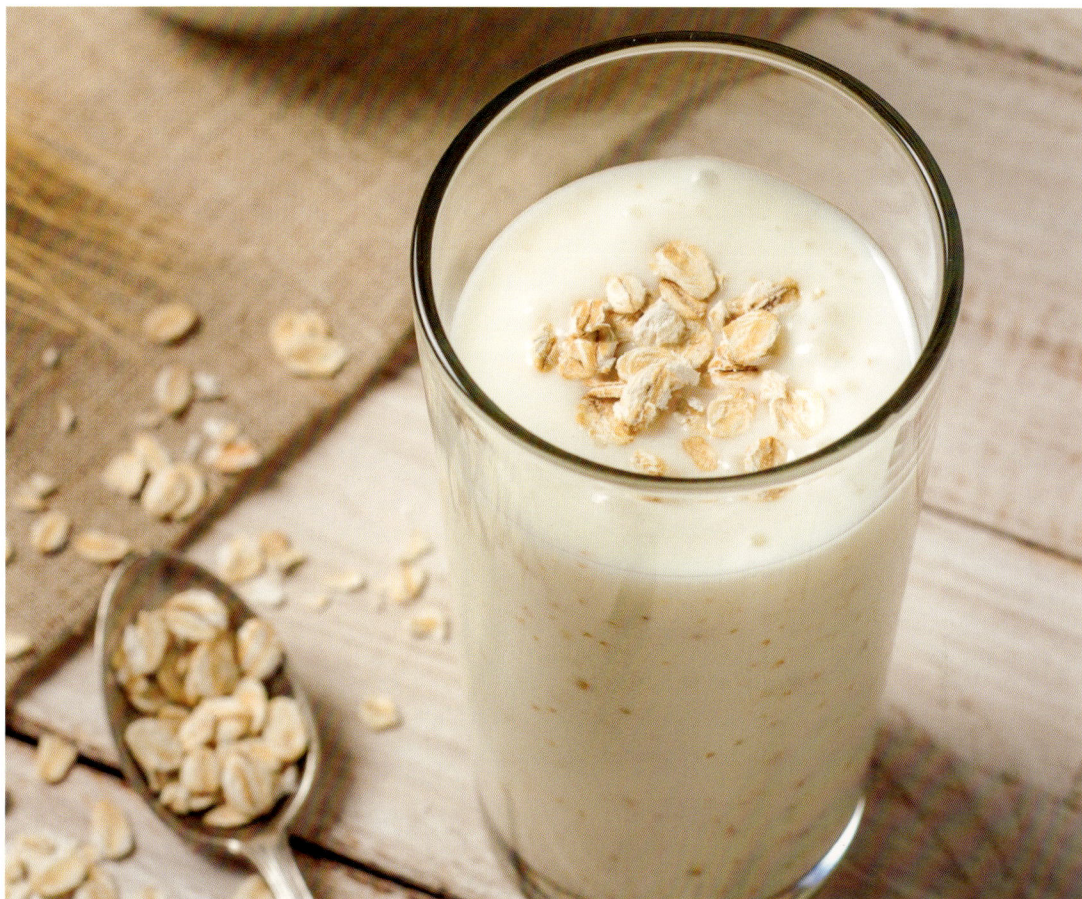

Apple Crisp Smoothie

TOTAL **5 MIN**. // SERVES **1**

Savor the taste of fall with this delicious smoothie, which features sweet apple cider, Greek yogurt, oats, nuts, and warming spices. It's also rich in protein and beta-glucan, a type of fiber that improves gut health.

1	**cup apple cider**
½	**cup 2% vanilla Greek yogurt**
¼	**cup old-fashioned rolled oats**
2	**Tbsp pecans**
¼	**tsp ground cinnamon**
¼	**tsp nutmeg**
1	**cup ice cubes**

In a blender, combine all ingredients and puree until smooth.

PER SERVING
410 cal, 14 g pro, 56 g carb, 3 g fiber, 38 g sugars (6 g added sugars), 14 g fat (3 g sat fat), 75 mg sodium

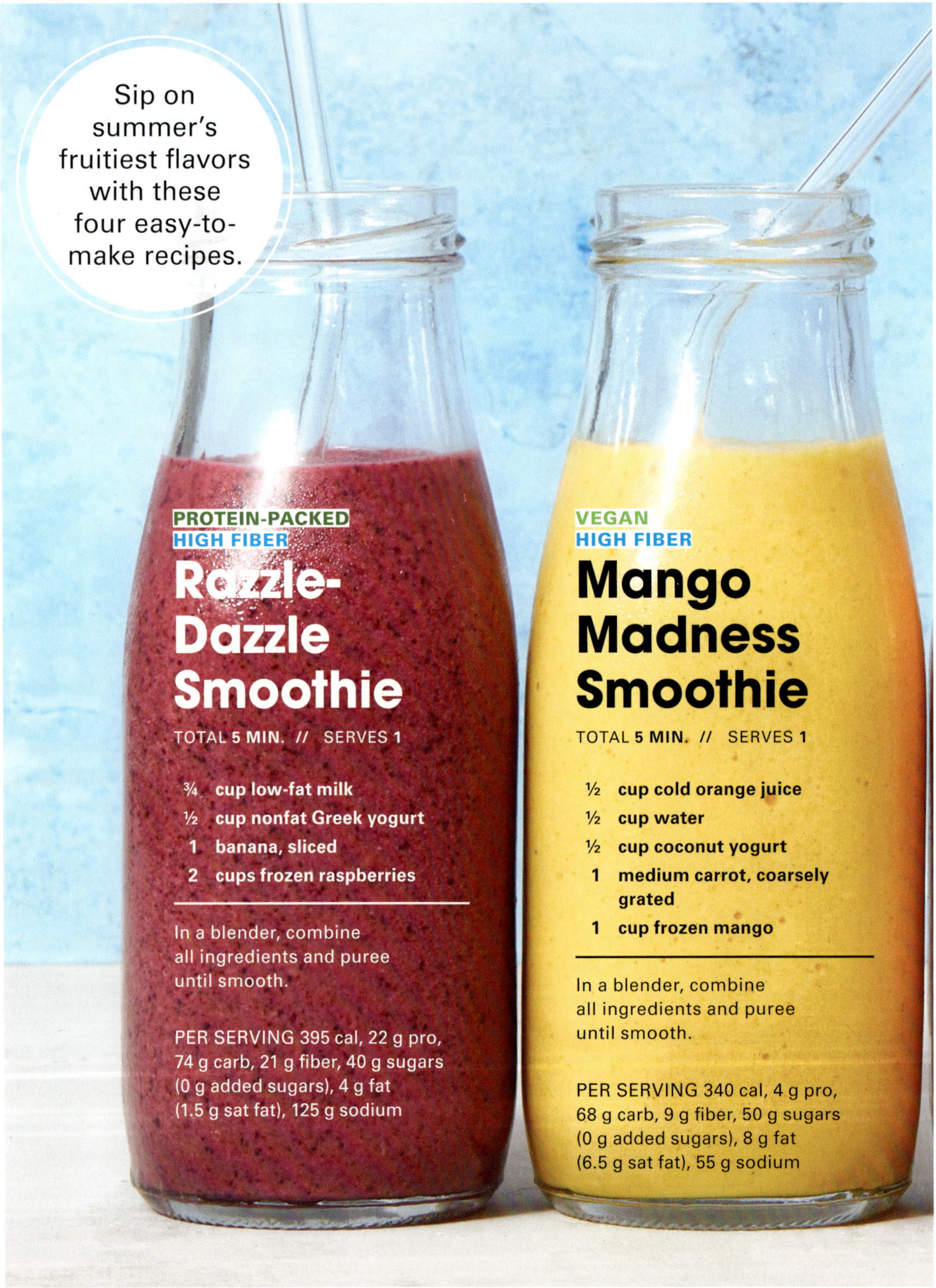

Sip on summer's fruitiest flavors with these four easy-to-make recipes.

PROTEIN-PACKED
HIGH FIBER

Razzle-Dazzle Smoothie

TOTAL **5 MIN.** // SERVES **1**

- ¾ cup low-fat milk
- ½ cup nonfat Greek yogurt
- 1 banana, sliced
- 2 cups frozen raspberries

In a blender, combine all ingredients and puree until smooth.

PER SERVING 395 cal, 22 g pro, 74 g carb, 21 g fiber, 40 g sugars (0 g added sugars), 4 g fat (1.5 g sat fat), 125 g sodium

VEGAN
HIGH FIBER

Mango Madness Smoothie

TOTAL **5 MIN.** // SERVES **1**

- ½ cup cold orange juice
- ½ cup water
- ½ cup coconut yogurt
- 1 medium carrot, coarsely grated
- 1 cup frozen mango

In a blender, combine all ingredients and puree until smooth.

PER SERVING 340 cal, 4 g pro, 68 g carb, 9 g fiber, 50 g sugars (0 g added sugars), 8 g fat (6.5 g sat fat), 55 g sodium

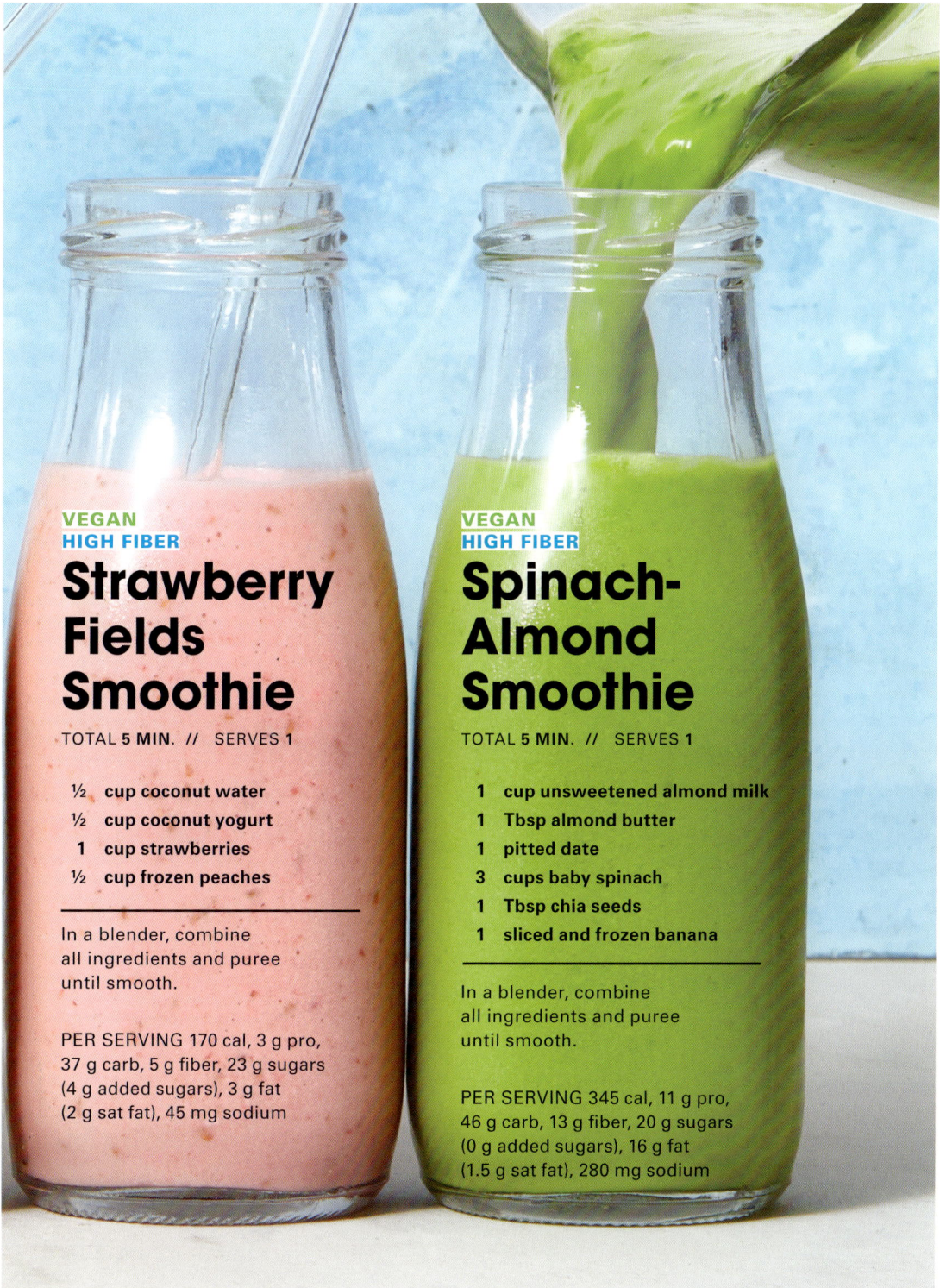

VEGAN
HIGH FIBER

Strawberry Fields Smoothie

TOTAL **5 MIN.** // SERVES **1**

½ cup coconut water
½ cup coconut yogurt
1 cup strawberries
½ cup frozen peaches

In a blender, combine all ingredients and puree until smooth.

PER SERVING 170 cal, 3 g pro, 37 g carb, 5 g fiber, 23 g sugars (4 g added sugars), 3 g fat (2 g sat fat), 45 mg sodium

VEGAN
HIGH FIBER

Spinach-Almond Smoothie

TOTAL **5 MIN.** // SERVES **1**

1 cup unsweetened almond milk
1 Tbsp almond butter
1 pitted date
3 cups baby spinach
1 Tbsp chia seeds
1 sliced and frozen banana

In a blender, combine all ingredients and puree until smooth.

PER SERVING 345 cal, 11 g pro, 46 g carb, 13 g fiber, 20 g sugars (0 g added sugars), 16 g fat (1.5 g sat fat), 280 mg sodium

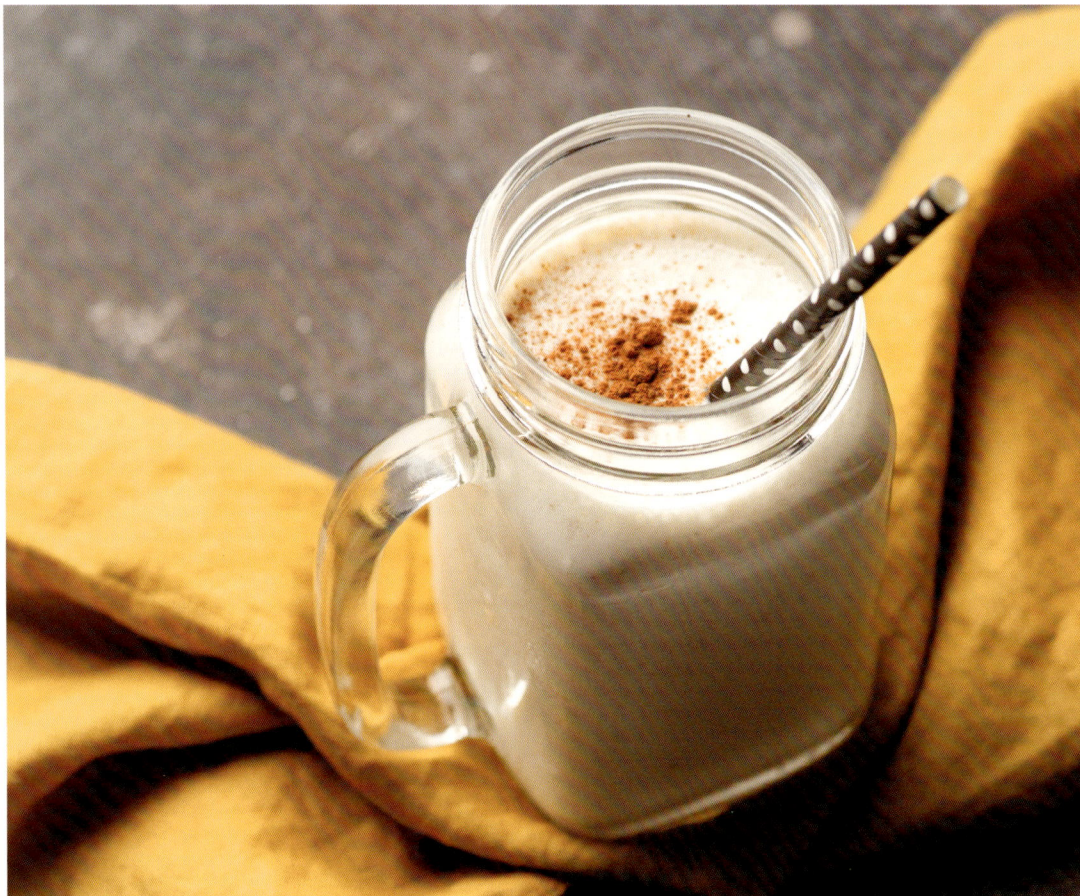

Cinnamon Spice

TOTAL **20 MIN**. // SERVES **1**

A little sprinkling of cinnamon goes a long way. This warm spice can do more than add an extra dose of cozy sweetness to any recipe—it contains polyphenol compounds that are thought to help with glucose control, which can keep type 2 diabetes at bay.

1½ **cups unsweetened almond or coconut milk**
1 **Tbsp honey**
¼ **cup raw cashews**
⅓ **cup rolled oats**
1 **tsp ground turmeric**
½ **tsp ground cinnamon**
½ **cup ice cubes**

1. Place cashews in a small bowl, cover with water and let soak for 15 min.; drain.

2. In a blender, puree cashews and remaining ingredients until smooth.

PER SERVING
390 cal, 10 g pro, 49 g carb, 6 g fiber, 19 g sugar (17 g added sugars), 19 g fat (3 g sat fat), 275 mg sodium

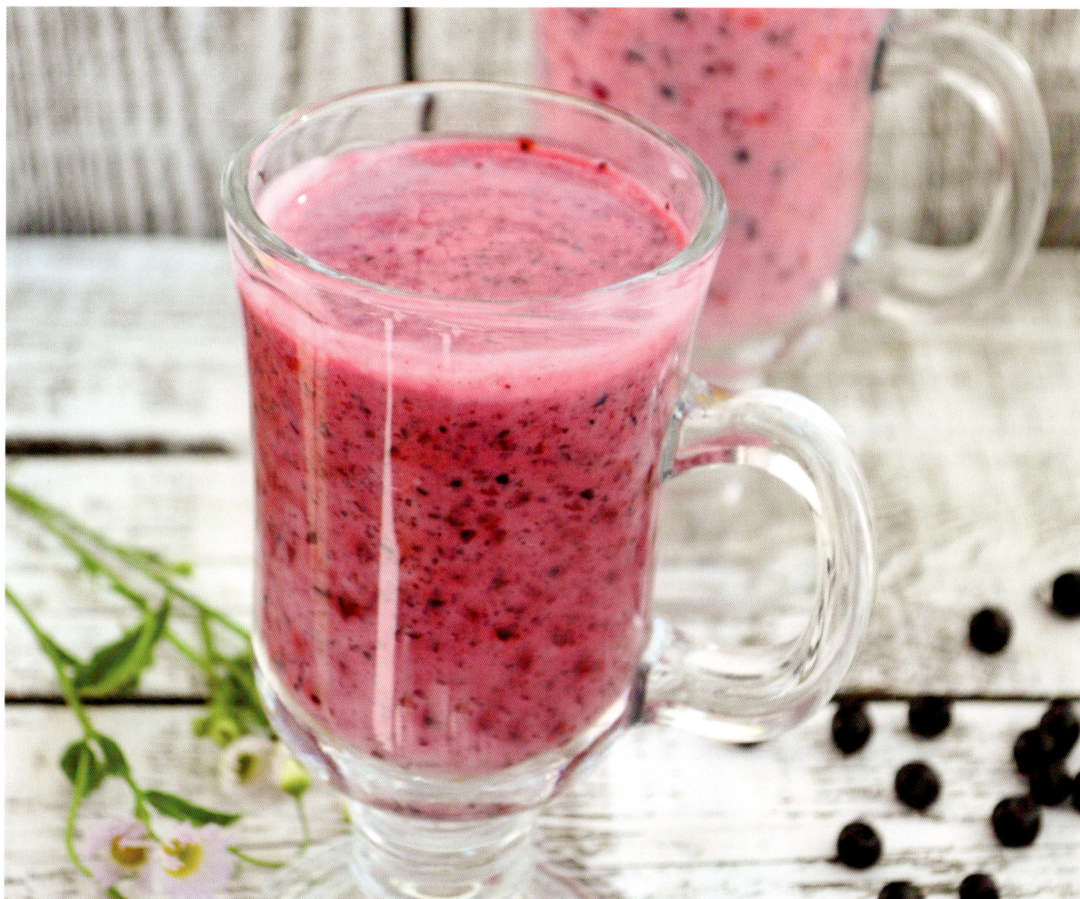

Mighty Cranberry Smoothie

HIGH FIBER

TOTAL **5 MIN**. // SERVES **1**

With a ton of advantages that range from preventing heart disease to protecting gums and staving off urinary tract infections, the bright-red cranberry is another superfood you wouldn't want to skimp on. Pair that with the anti-inflammatory properties of pineapple and the probiotic powers of yogurt, and you get a potent combo of nutrients that help keep your immune system in tip-top shape.

½ **cup unsweetened cranberry juice**

6 **oz low-fat plain, vanilla, or berry yogurt**

½ **cup blueberries**

1 **banana**

½ **cup fresh or frozen cranberries**

½ **cup fresh or frozen pineapple chunks**

In a blender, combine all ingredients and puree until smooth.

PER SERVING
375 cal, 12 g pro, 82 g carb, 8 g fiber, 59 g sugars (0 g added sugars), 4 g fat (2 g sat fat), 125 mg sodium

Go Grape Smoothie

TOTAL **5 MIN**. // SERVES **1**

Grapes are naturally a low-calorie, fat-free food with a relatively low glycemic index. We threw them into this smoothie along with heart-healthy cashews, potassium-packed bananas, and fiber- and iron-rich spinach for a nutrient-dense glass of goodness.

- **1   cup unsweetened cashew milk**
- **2   Tbsp almond butter**
- **1   cup spinach**
- **1   banana**
- **1   Tbsp ground flaxseed**
- **½   cup frozen red seedless grapes**

In a blender, combine all ingredients and puree until smooth.

PER SERVING 425 cal, 10 g pro, 50 g carb, 9 g fiber, 28 g sugars (0 g added sugars), 24 g fat (2.5 g sat fat), 90 mg sodium

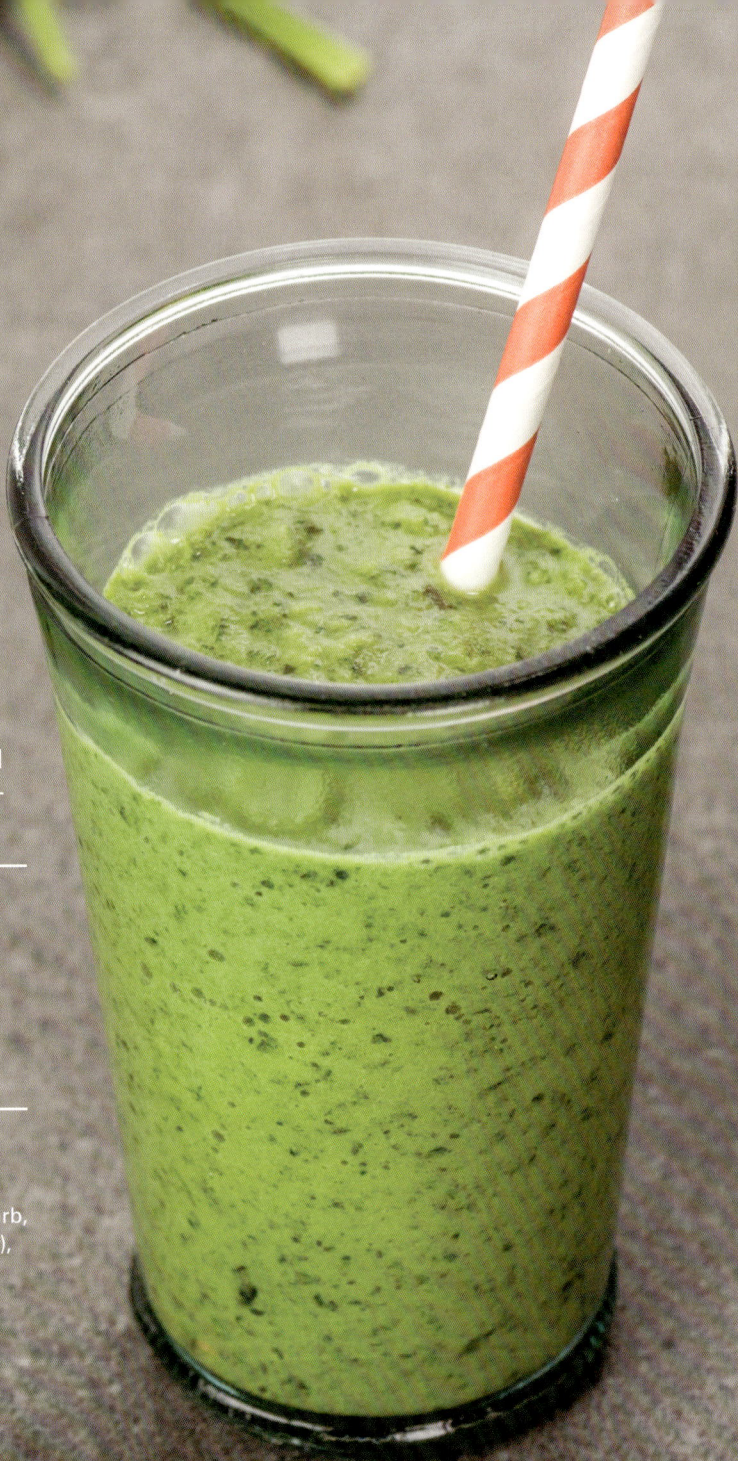

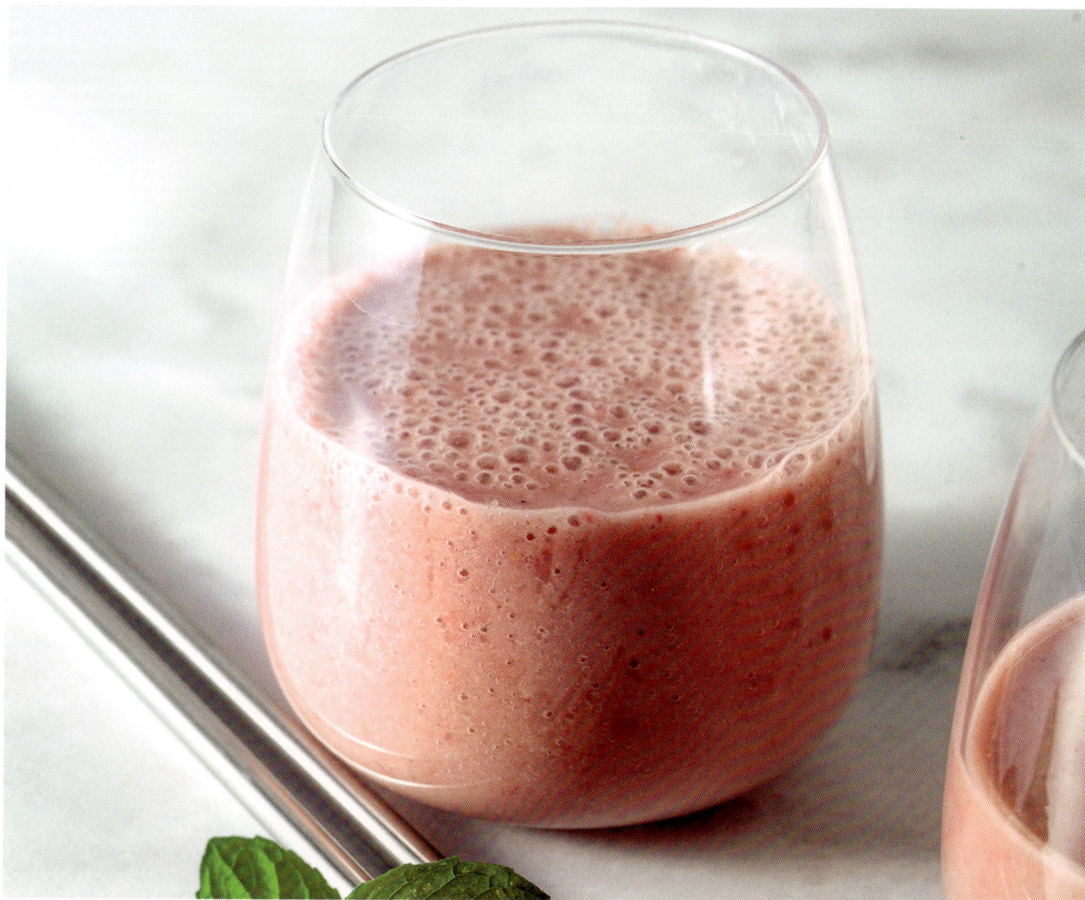

Peachy Keen

TOTAL **5 MIN.** // SERVES **1**

Peaches, strawberries, and orange juice are the heroes in this blended treat. All are high in vitamin C to support a healthy body. We added yogurt packed with probiotics and good bacteria to keep your gut healthy, which is hugely beneficial for your immunity and digestion.

1	**cup fresh orange juice**
6	**oz peach-flavored 2% Greek yogurt**
1	**cup frozen sliced peaches**
1	**cup frozen strawberries**
½	**cup frozen pineapple chunks**

In a blender, combine all ingredients and puree until smooth.

PER SERVING
415 cal, 15 g pro,
86 g carb, 7 g fiber,
69 g sugars (12 g
added sugars),
4 g fat (2 g sat fat),
50 mg sodium

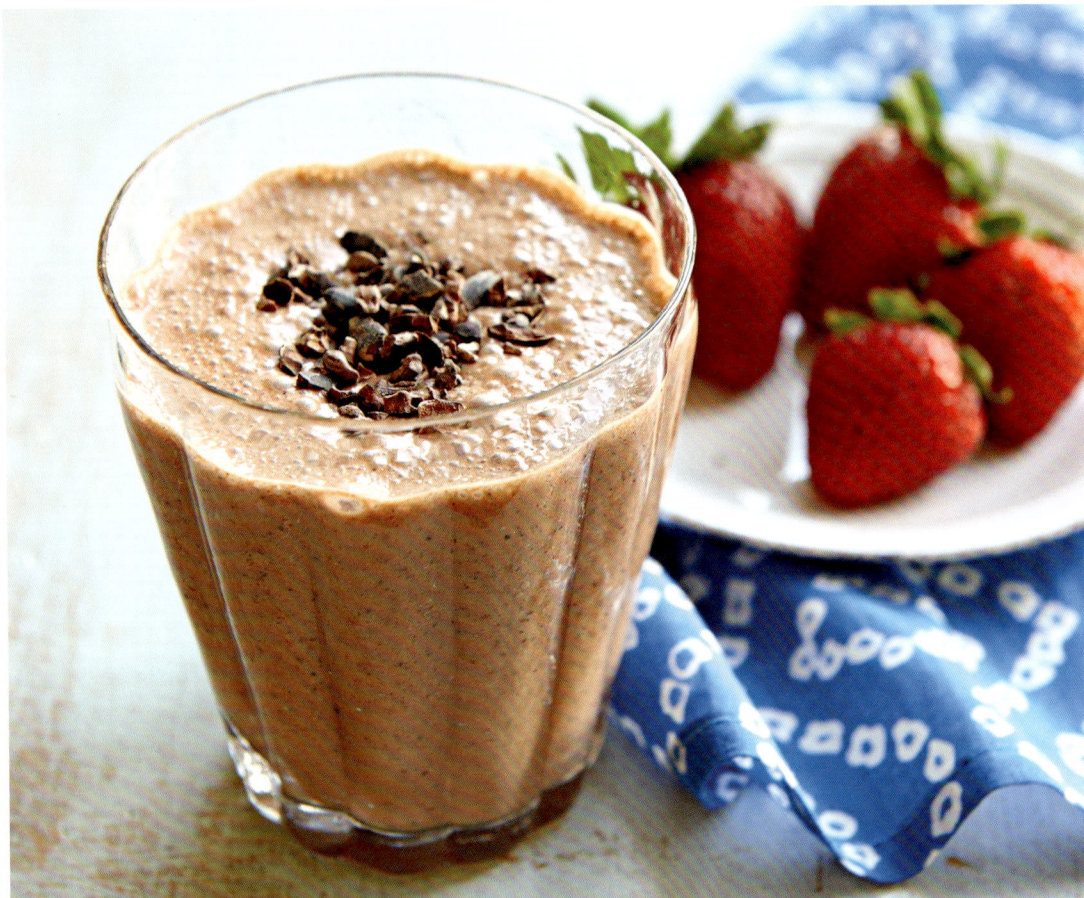

Heart-Smart Chocolate Berry HIGH FIBER

TOTAL **5 MIN**. // SERVES **1**

Yogurt contains beneficial lactobacillus bacteria that can help keep you regular and reduce gut inflammation triggered by overindulgence in sugary foods and alcohol. All that in a blend of creamy goodness!

1 **cup unsweetened almond or coconut milk**

½ **cup plain 2% Greek yogurt**

2 **Tbsp cacao nibs, plus more for serving, optional**

1 **Tbsp unsweetened cocoa powder**

1 **cup frozen strawberries**

In a blender, combine all ingredients and puree until smooth. Sprinkle more cacao nibs on top, if desired.

PER SERVING
260 cal, 13 g pro, 30 g carb, 10 g fiber, 13 g sugars (0 g added sugars), 12 g fat (4 g sat fat), 240 mg sodium

Cherry-Chia Smoothie

TOTAL **10 MIN**. // SERVES **1**

It's not always easy to get the recommended 25 to 30 grams of fiber per day. But with 3 grams of fiber per cup, cherries are a delicious way to get closer to your goal—and reap the benefits that come with it. Fiber-rich foods have been shown to aid in healthy body weight, improved gut health, and lower risk of heart disease.

¾ **cup unsweetened almond or coconut milk**

2 **kiwis, peeled and chopped**

1 **Tbsp chia seeds**

1 **Tbsp ground ginger**

1 **cup frozen cherries, pitted**

In a blender, combine all ingredients and puree until smooth.

PER SERVING
260 cal, 5 g pro, 49 g carb, 12 g fiber, 31 g sugars (0 g added sugars) 6 g fat (0 g sat fat), 140 mg sodium

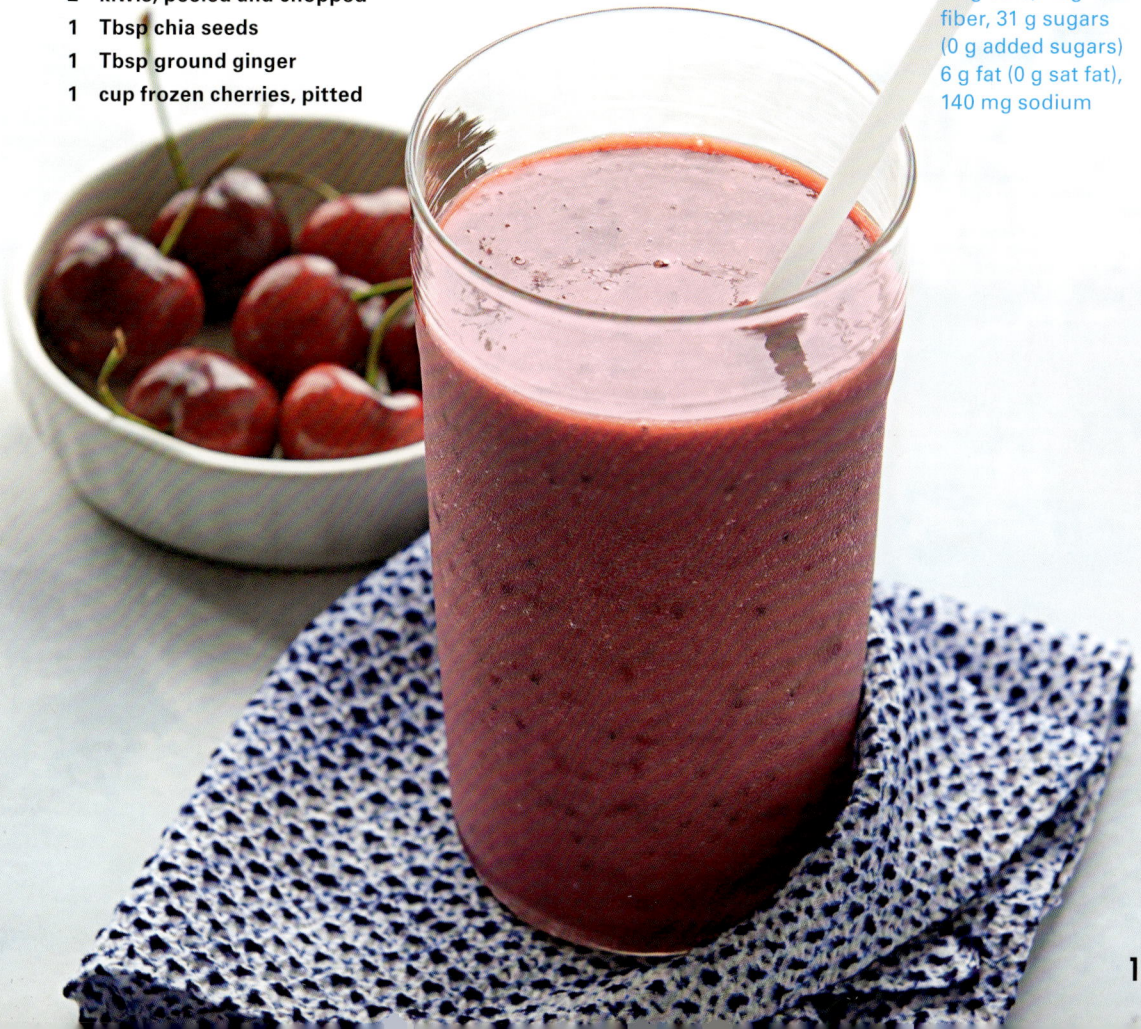

Pineapple-Pear Smoothie

TOTAL **10 MIN**. // SERVES **1**

This smoothie is a perfect example of how easy it is to turn your salad into a delicious drink you can have on the go. The natural sweetness of pears and pineapples balances out the slight bitterness that kale or romaine lettuce may have for a perfect blend that packs a whopping 13 grams of fiber.

- 1 **cup coconut water**
- 1 **small pear, seeded and cut into pieces**
- 1 **lemon, peeled, seeded, and chopped**
- 1 **cup spinach or kale**
- 3 **leaves romaine lettuce**
- 4 **sprigs parsley**
- 2 **Tbsp ground flaxseed**
- ½ **cup frozen pineapple chunks**

In a blender, combine all ingredients and puree until smooth.

PER SERVING 275 cal, 6 g pro, 56 g carb, 13 g fiber, 29 g sugars (0 g added sugars), 6.5 g fat (0.5 g sat fat), 95 mg sodium

Melon-Berry Smoothie

TOTAL **5 MIN**. // SERVES **1**

Watermelon is one of the richest sources of the amino acid citrulline, which opens veins and arteries to improve blood flow and reduce blood pressure. That helps keep arteries clear and leads to improved circulation and overall cardiovascular health. This summery smoothie also blends in chia seeds—an excellent source of omega-3 fatty acids, which help to raise HDL ("good") cholesterol levels.

- 5.3 **-oz vanilla plant-based yogurt**
- 1 **Tbsp lime juice**
- ½ **tsp agave or honey, to taste**
- 2 **cups watermelon chunks**
- 1 **Tbsp chia seeds**
- 1 **cup frozen strawberries**

In a blender, combine all ingredients and puree until smooth.

PER SERVING 300 cal, 8 g pro, 65 g carb, 9 g fiber, 38 g sugars (5 g added sugars), 7.5 g fat (0.5 g sat fat), 50 mg sodium

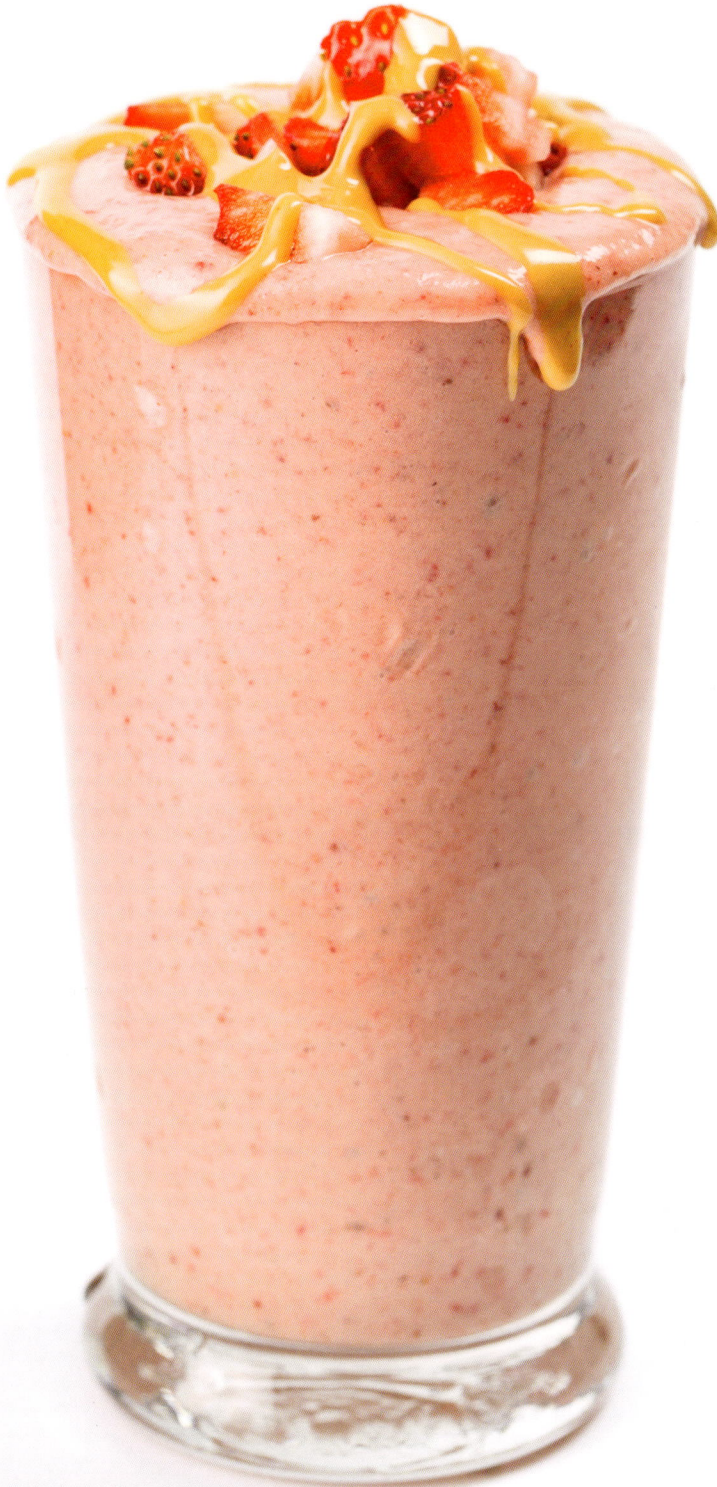

PB&J Smoothie

TOTAL **5 MIN**. // SERVES **1**

It may seem counterintuitive to call your favorite childhood sandwich in smoothie form a diet food. But this smoothie combines the high fiber in strawberries with the protein in peanut butter to keep you feeling full longer, so you eat less overall. Go ahead, indulge a little!

---

1   cup skim milk

¼   cup peanut butter, plus more for garnish

1   banana

2   Tbsp fresh strawberries, chopped

1   cup frozen strawberries

In a blender, combine all ingredients and puree until smooth. Pour into a glass and garnish with peanut butter and fresh strawberries.

PER SERVING 770 cal, 28 g pro, 69 g carb, 12 g fiber, 37 g sugars (0 g added sugars), 41 g fat (6.5 g sat fat), 370 mg sodium

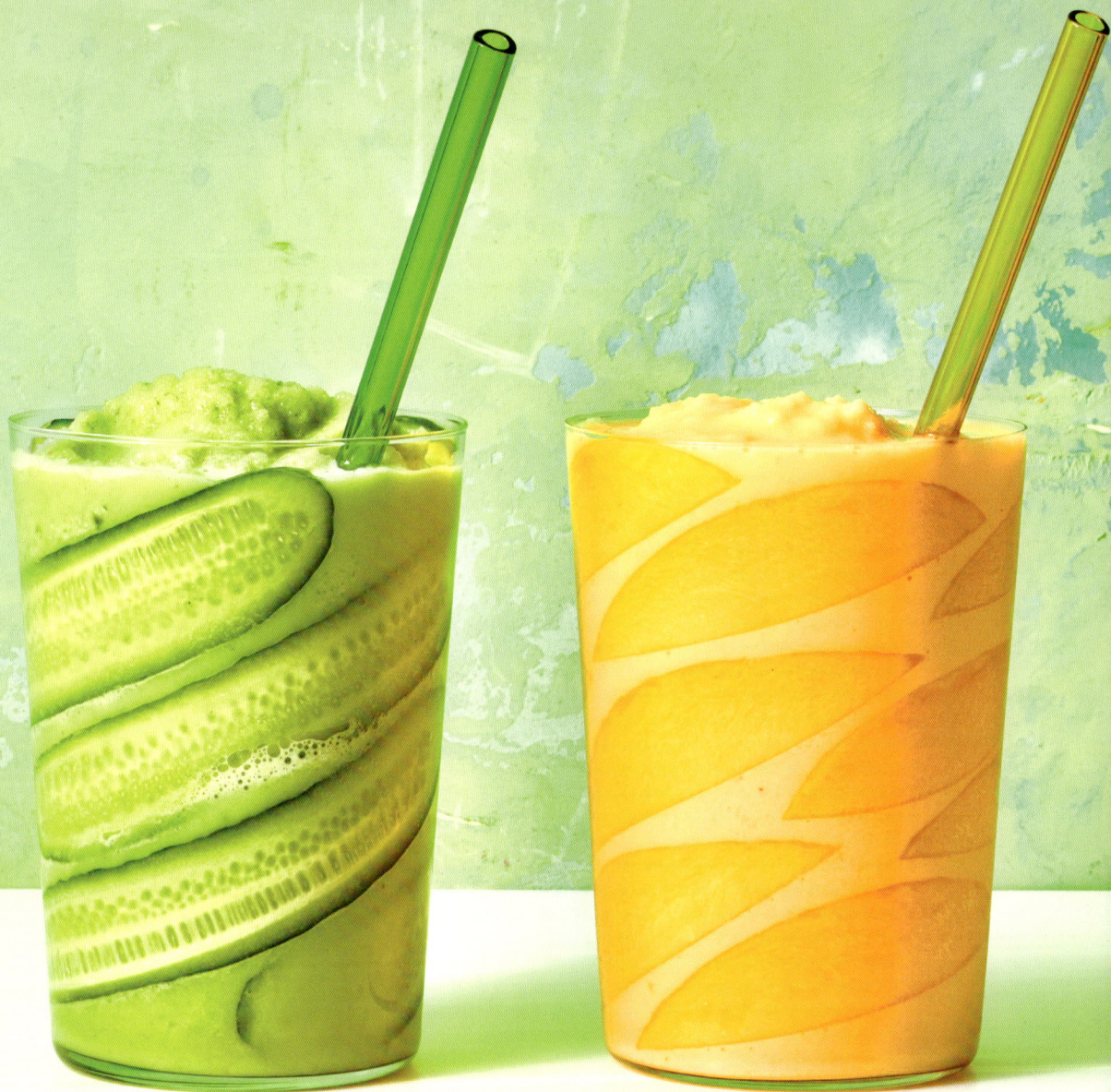

HIGH FIBER **PROTEIN-PACKED**

Pineapple-Cucumber Smoothie

TOTAL **5 MIN**. // SERVES **1**

Bright and refreshing, this cooling smoothie is perfect for a hot summer's day.

¼   **cup unsweetened almond milk**
½   **cup plain Greek yogurt**
1   **Tbsp fresh lemon juice**
1   **Persian cucumber, chopped**
1   **frozen banana, halved**
1   **cup frozen pineapple chunks**
1   **cup baby spinach**

In a blender, combine all ingredients and puree until smooth.

PER SERVING 360 cal, 16 g pro, 62 g carb, 8 g fiber, 25 g sugars (0 g added sugars), 8 g fat (3 g sat fat), 120 mg sodium

HIGH FIBER

Peach-Mango Smoothie

TOTAL **5 MIN**. // SERVES **1**

This springy smoothie provides ample hydration after yoga or a power walk with your pup.

⅓   **cup coconut water**
½   **cup plain Greek yogurt**
1   **cup frozen sliced peaches**
1   **cup frozen mango chunks**

In a blender, combine all ingredients and puree until smooth.

PER SERVING 310 cal, 14 g pro, 52 g carb, 6 g fiber, 47 g sugars (0 g added sugars), 6 g fat (3 g sat fat), 70 mg sodium

All-Around Health Booster

TOTAL **5 MIN.** // SERVES **1**

Fight inflammation and help protect cells from damage with pomegranate's antioxidants. Combine with potassium-rich foods (to support blood pressure) and fiber (for gut health) and you've got yourself a delicious health boost.

- ⅓ cup almond milk
- ⅓ cup plain Greek yogurt
- ¾ cup pomegranate juice
- ½ tsp honey
- 1 banana

In a blender, combine all ingredients and puree until smooth.

PER SERVING 325 cal, 10 g pro, 63 g carb, 3 g fiber, 45 g sugars (3 g added sugars), 5.5 g fat (2 g sat fat), 90 mg sodium

Watermelon Smoothie

TOTAL **5 MIN.** // SERVES **1**

Watermelon and raspberries combine to make the most refreshing summer drink. Sub in any berry you have around, but don't skip the chia seeds, which help make this a smoothie that will actually fill you up.

- ½ cup plain Greek yogurt
- 1 Tbsp lime juice
- 3 cups chopped watermelon (about 1 lb)
- ½ cup frozen raspberries
- 1 Tbsp chia seeds

In a blender, combine all ingredients and puree until smooth. Add chia seeds and blend on low until incorporated, but still whole.

PER SERVING 335 cal, 16 g pro, 60 g carb, 11 g fiber, 46 g sugars (0 g added sugars), 10 g fat (3.5 g sat fat), 60 mg sodium

Cranberry-Banana Smoothie

TOTAL 5 MIN. // SERVES 1

The autumn berry is the star of this satisfying, fiber-rich treat. Potassium in bananas helps regulate the balance of fluids in your body, and yogurt packs in the protein. Blend it all together to make this great post-workout recovery drink.

¾	cup unsweetened almond milk
½	cup vanilla yogurt
1	Tbsp maple syrup
1	banana, sliced
1	cup frozen cranberries
½	cup ice cubes

In a blender, combine all ingredients and puree until smooth.

PER SERVING 350 cal, 9 g pro, 70 g carb, 7 g fiber, 47 g sugars (20 g added sugars), 6.5 g fat (3 g sat fat), 220 mg sodium

VEGAN   HIGH FIBER
PROTEIN-PACKED

Quick Breakfast Smoothie

TOTAL **5 MIN.** // SERVES **1**

For instant energy without feeling full, turn to the natural sugars of orange juice. It also contains electrolytes that help prevent muscle cramps. Blend it up with some muscle-building protein powder and gut-friendly probiotics from yogurt for an ideal preworkout fuel.

- 1 **cup calcium-fortified orange juice**
- 6 **oz low-fat vanilla yogurt**
- 1 **banana**
- 2 **tsp protein powder (preferably plant-based)**
- 1 **cup frozen raspberries**
- ¼ **cup ice**

In a blender, combine all ingredients and puree until smooth.

PER SERVING 450 cal, 16 g pro, 96 g carb, 13 g fiber, 65 g sugars (14 g added sugars), 4 g fat (1.5 g sat fat), 125 mg sodium

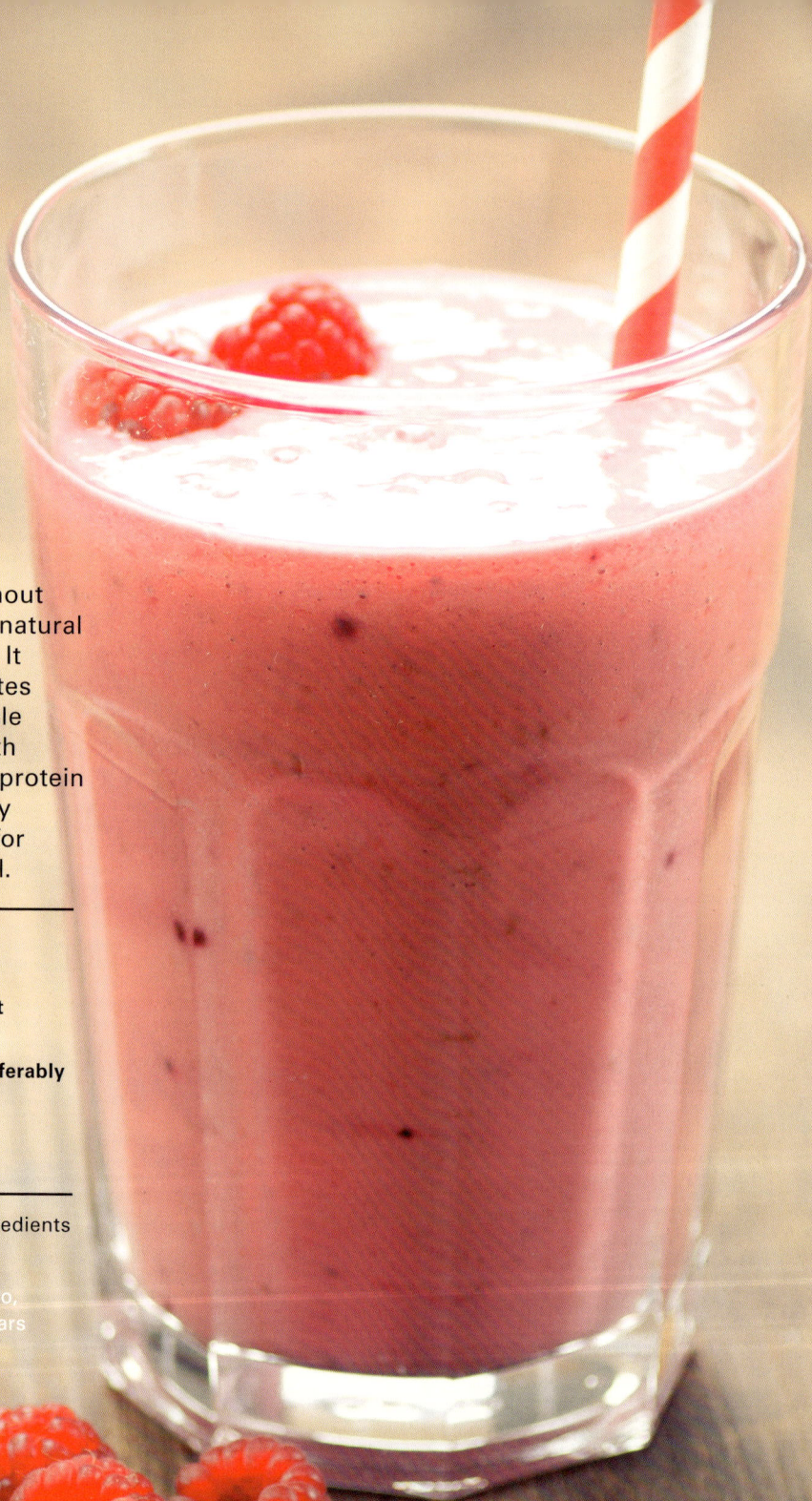

Mocha Protein Shake

TOTAL **5 MIN.** // SERVES **1**

This buzzy breakfast tastes like a milkshake. The secret ingredient? Walnuts, which are high in protein and omega-3 fatty acids—healthy fats known to help fight inflammation and protect your heart. A dose of black coffee makes this the perfect morning shake.

- ¾ **cup cold black coffee**
- 2 **Tbsp walnuts**
- ½ **Tbsp unsweetened cocoa powder**
- 3 **Tbsp chocolate protein powder**
- ½ **large banana, sliced and frozen**
- ½ **cup ice**

In a blender, combine all ingredients and puree until smooth.

PER SERVING 285 cal, 19 g pro, 30 g carb, 7 g fiber, 10 g sugars (0 g added sugars), 12.5 g fat (2 g sat fat), 260 mg sodium

Green Tea, Blueberry, and Banana Smoothie

TOTAL **10 MIN.** // SERVES **1**

Brew some antioxidant-rich green tea to help boost metabolism and burn fat. Pair it with blueberries, bananas, and light vanilla soy milk for a filling breakfast that's sure to start your day right.

- 1 **green tea bag**
- ½ **tsp honey**
- ¾ **cup calcium-fortified vanilla soy milk**
- ½ **medium banana, sliced**
- 1½ **cups frozen blueberries**

---

1. Heat 3 Tbsp water in a bowl in the microwave until it's steaming hot.

2. Add tea bag and allow to brew for 3 min. Remove the tea bag and stir in honey until it dissolves.

3. In a blender, puree tea and remaining ingredients until smooth.

PER SERVING 245 cal, 7 g pro, 52 g carb, 9 g fiber, 31 g sugars (3 g added sugars), 3 g fat (0.5 g sat fat), 120 mg sodium

VEGAN HIGH FIBER

Healthy-Up Your Tummy

TOTAL **5 MIN.** // SERVES **1**

You might think it's odd to put thyme in your smoothie, but the herb's antioxidant properties may soothe digestive muscles, relieving gas and bloating. Thyme is also reputed to support a healthy mix of gut bacteria, making it an ideal partner to antioxidant-rich blueberries in aiding weight management.

1½	cups unsweetened almond milk
1	Tbsp almond butter
	Leaves from 3 thyme sprigs
1	banana, frozen
1	cup blueberries, fresh or frozen

In a blender, combine all ingredients and puree until smooth.

PER SERVING 350 cal, 7 g pro, 55 g carb, 10 g fiber, 30 g sugars (0 g added sugars), 15 g fat (1.5 g sat fat), 275 mg sodium

VEGAN HIGH FIBER

Mango-Peach Batido

TOTAL **5 MIN.** // SERVES **1**

Batidos are Latino smoothies or milkshakes. We used coconut milk in this recipe to add a natural sweetness for relatively fewer calories, and paired it with mangoes and peaches for a tropical smoothie you can enjoy all year-round.

⅓	cup water
¼	cup coconut milk
2	Tbsp fresh lime juice
1	cup frozen mango pieces
1	cup frozen sliced peaches
¼	cup ice cubes

In blender, combine all ingredients and puree until smooth.

PER SERVING 285 cal, 3 g pro, 48 g carb, 6 g fiber, 40 g sugars (0 g added sugars), 12 g fat (10.5 g sat fat), 10 mg sodium

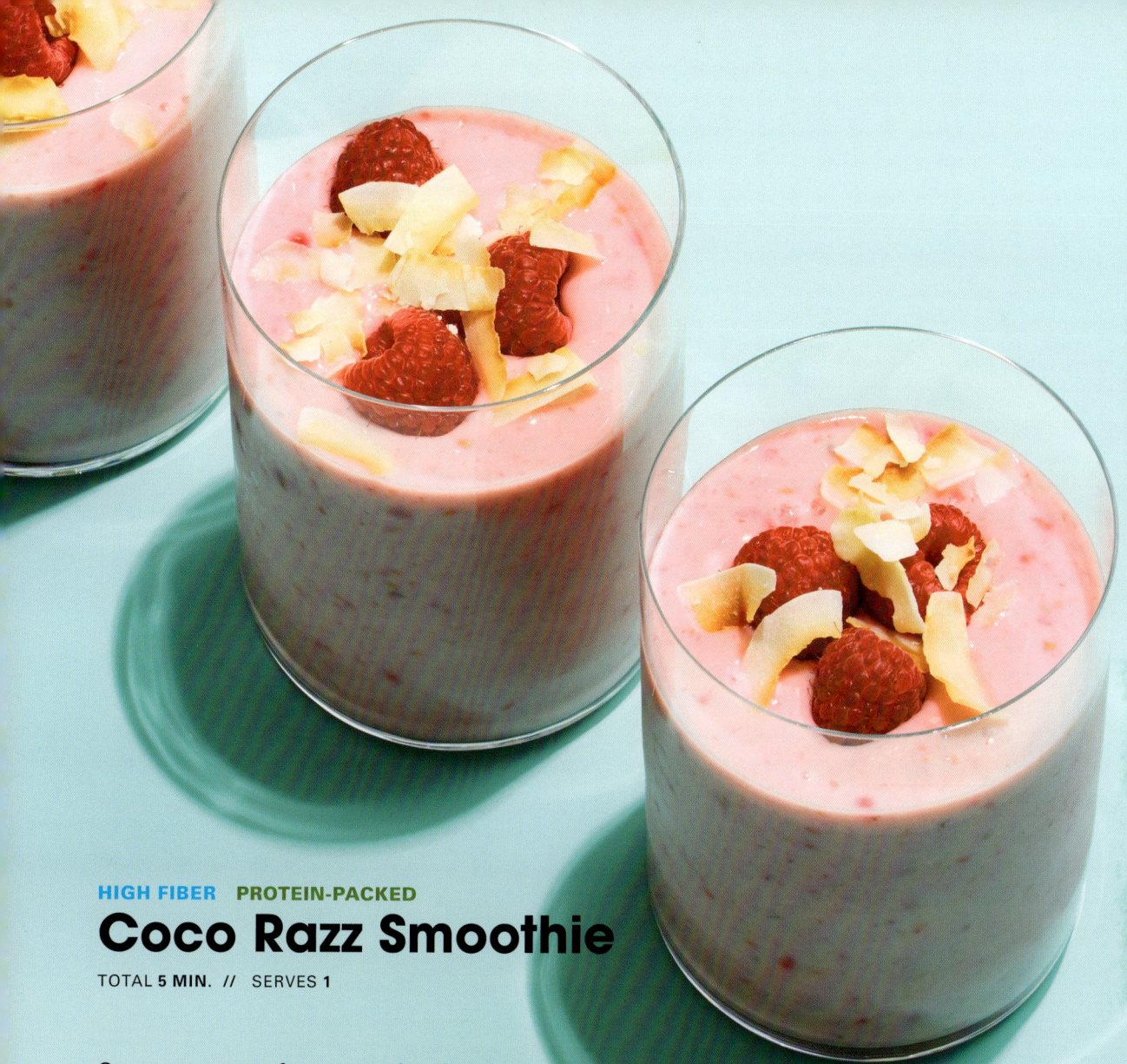

HIGH FIBER   PROTEIN-PACKED

Coco Razz Smoothie

TOTAL **5 MIN.** // SERVES **1**

Coconut yogurt, frozen raspberries, and bananas create a creamy and fiber-rich breakfast or snack treat.

½ cup low-fat milk

½ cup low-fat coconut-flavored yogurt

1 banana

2 cup frozen raspberries

Toasted coconut, for serving

Fresh raspberries, for serving

In a blender, combine all ingredients and puree until smooth. Serve garnished with coconut and raspberries.

PER SERVING
410 cal, 15 g pro, 82 g carb, 21 g fiber, 47 g sugars (6 g added sugars), 5 g fat (2 g sat fat), 150 mg sodium

Superfruit Smoothie

TOTAL **5 MIN.** // SERVES **1**

While a fraction of the size of an orange, a single kiwi has as much vitamin C and fiber and is among the few low-fat sources of vitamin E (10% of the RDA), all for about 50 calories. Mixed with antioxidant-rich cherries and satiety-boosting chia seeds, this smoothie will have you feeling full and eating less in the long run.

- ½ **cup almond milk**
- ½ **Tbsp chia seeds**
- ½ **kiwi, peeled and sliced, plus more slices for serving**
- ½ **cup frozen cherries**

In a blender, combine all ingredients and puree until smooth. Serve with kiwi slices, if desired.

PER SERVING 115 cal, 2 g pro, 19 g carb, 5 g fiber, 12 g sugars (0 g added sugars), 3.5 g fat (0.5 g sat fat), 90 mg sodium

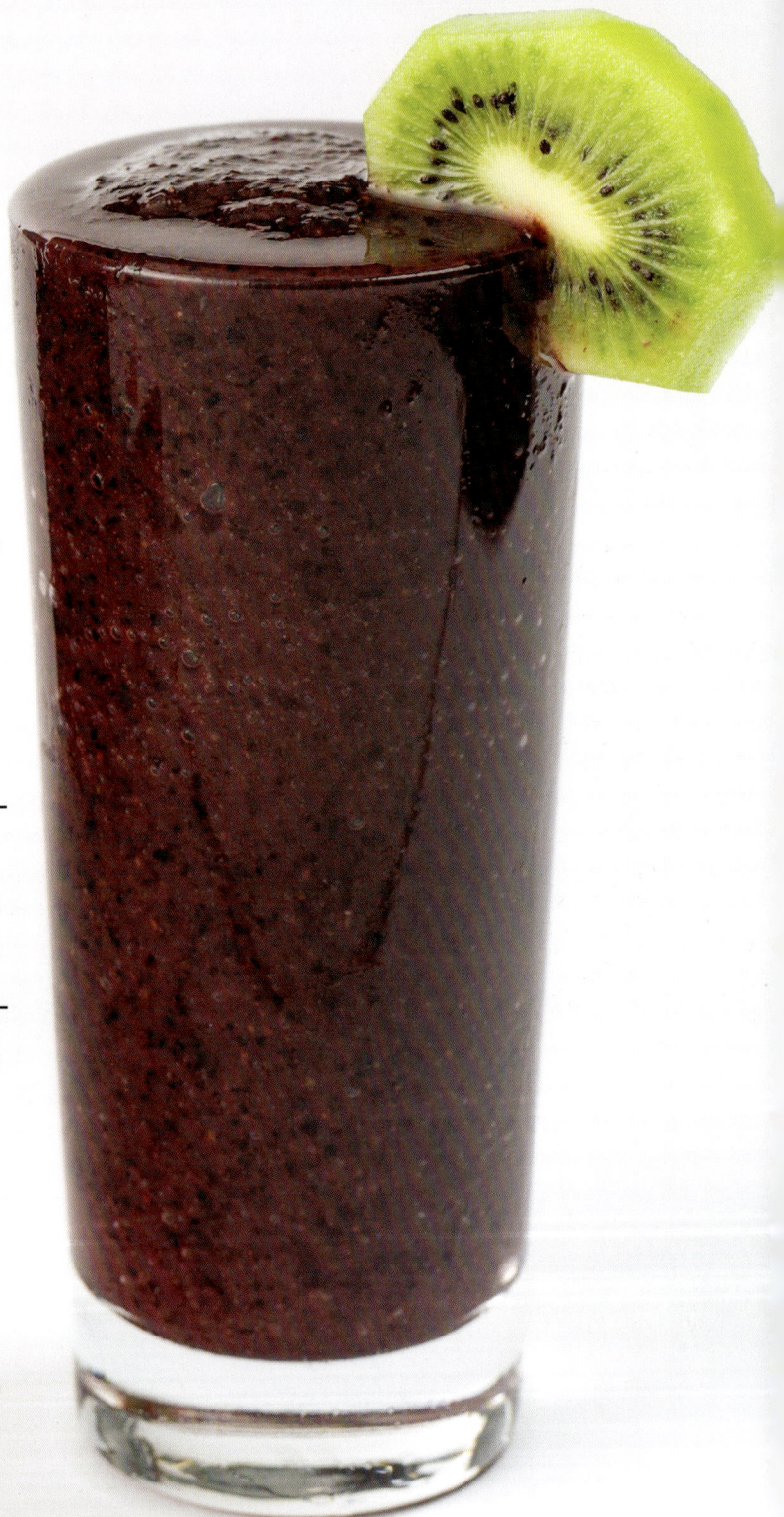

Three-Berry Smoothie

TOTAL **5 MIN.** // SERVES **1**

Using a frozen berry medley lets you get to enjoy the summery taste of berries— along with all their health benefits—all year-round.

½ **cup cranberry-raspberry juice, refrigerated**

½ **cup low-fat vanilla yogurt**

1 **cup frozen berry medley (strawberries, raspberries, blackberries, and blueberries)**

In a blender, combine all ingredients and puree until smooth.

PER SERVING 280 cal, 9 g pro, 53 g carb, 8 g fiber, 39 g sugars (25 g added sugars), 3 g fat (1 g sat fat), 85 g sodium

Strawberry Blast

TOTAL **5 MIN.** // SERVES **1**

The high fiber content of strawberries helps control cravings; plus, they're super low in calories. The yogurt offers protein to help fill you up.

¼ **cup cranberry juice cocktail, chilled**

1 **8-oz container low-fat strawberry yogurt**

1 **cup frozen strawberries**

In blender, combine all ingredients and puree until smooth.

PER SERVING 260 cal, 7 g pro, 53 g carb, 3 g fiber, 40 g sugars (16 g added sugars), 2 g fat (1.5 g sat fat), 90 mg sodium

Mango-Go-Go

TOTAL **5 MIN**. // SERVES **1**

Orange fruits and veggies offer heaps of nutrients called carotenoids, which repair the cell damage that happens during workouts. Meanwhile, coconut water rebalances the electrolytes you've lost through perspiration.

2	**cups baby spinach**
1	**cup frozen mango chunks**
½	**cup shredded carrots**
½	**cup coconut water**
¼	**cup orange juice**
2	**satsuma or mandarin oranges, peeled**
½	**cup low-fat plain yogurt**

In a blender, combine all ingredients and puree until smooth.

PER SERVING 365 cal, 12 g pro, 80 g carb, 12 g fiber, 62 g sugars (0 g added sugars), 2.5 g fat (1.5 g sat fat), 320 mg sodium

Creamy Banana-Blueberry Smoothie

TOTAL **5 MIN**. // SERVES **1**

Succulent blueberries are bursting with flavor in this healthy smoothie, which is also loaded with potassium-rich banana and vanilla for sweetness.

1	**cup oat milk**
1	**tsp pure vanilla extract**
1	**Tbsp almond butter**
1	**banana, sliced and frozen**
¾	**cup frozen blueberries**

In a blender, combine all ingredients and puree until smooth.

PER SERVING 310 cal, 6 g pro, 46 g carb, 8 g fiber, 24 g sugars (0 g added sugars), 12.5 g fat (1 g sat fat), 110 mg sodium

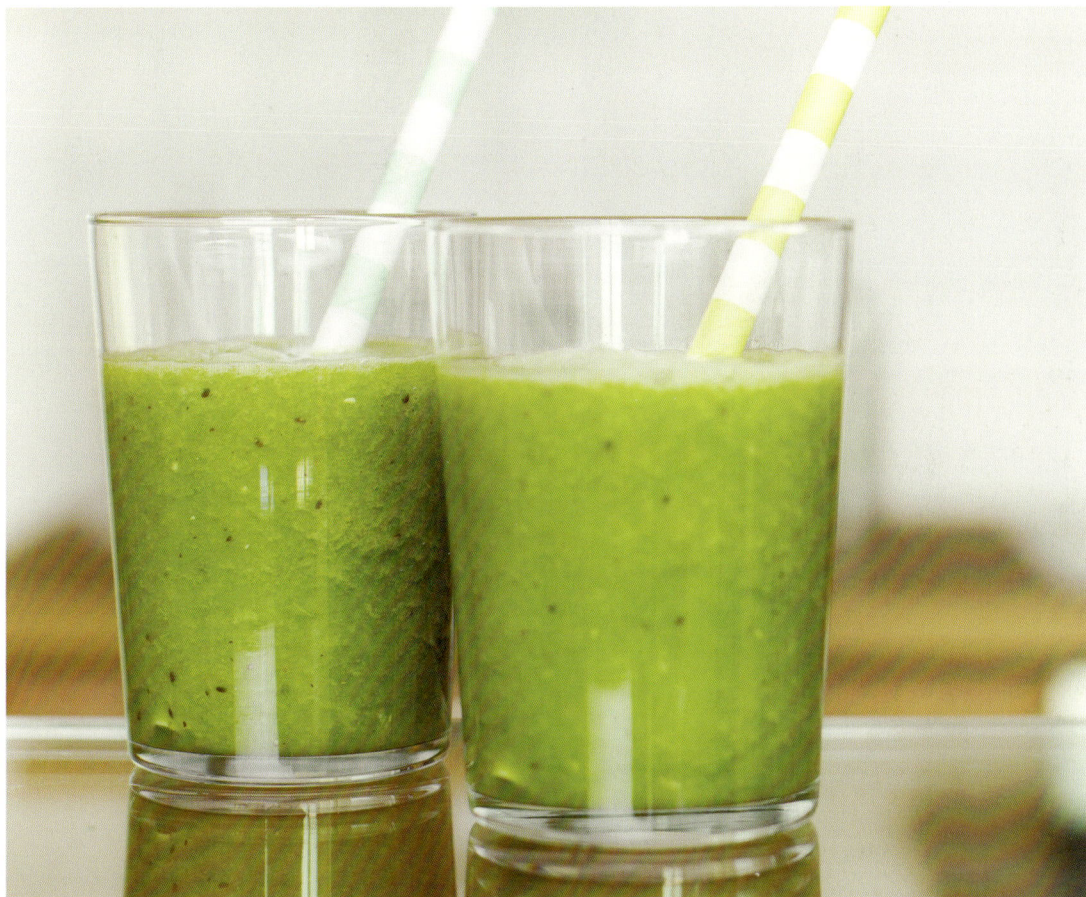

Green Tea Wakeup

HIGH FIBER

TOTAL **10 MIN**. // SERVES **1**

A perfect alternative to your morning joe, green tea has enough caffeine to keep you energized and alert for whatever the day brings. Combined with honeydew and avocado, it makes a refreshingly delicious smoothie that just could become addictive!

¼ **cup unsweetened almond or cashew milk**

¾ **cup brewed green tea (use 2 tea bags and steep for 10 min. to make it strong)**

½ **tsp honey**

2 **cups chopped honeydew melon**

1 **small avocado (or half a large), peeled and seeded**

In a blender, combine all ingredients and puree until smooth.

PER SERVING
390 cal, 6 g pro, 47 g carb, 13 g fiber, 52 g sugars (3 g added sugars), 23 g fat (3.5 g sat fat), 120 mg sodium

Avocado Mint

TOTAL **10 MIN**. // SERVES **1**

Mint not only smells great; it's a soothing herb that can help ease an upset stomach. Mint increases bile secretion and encourages bile flow, which speeds and eases digestion. When you combine it with the bromelain found in pineapple, you've got a refreshing smoothie that tastes great, settles an upset tummy quickly, and boosts digestive health.

1	cup coconut water
¼	cup chopped parsley
6	fresh mint leaves
1	tsp grated fresh ginger
1	avocado, peeled and seeded
1	large banana, frozen
½	cup frozen pineapple chunks

In a blender, combine all ingredients and puree until smooth.

PER SERVING 540 cal, 7 g pro, 72 g carb, 19 g fiber, 30 g sugars (0 g added sugars), 30 g fat (4.5 g sat fat), 90 mg sodium

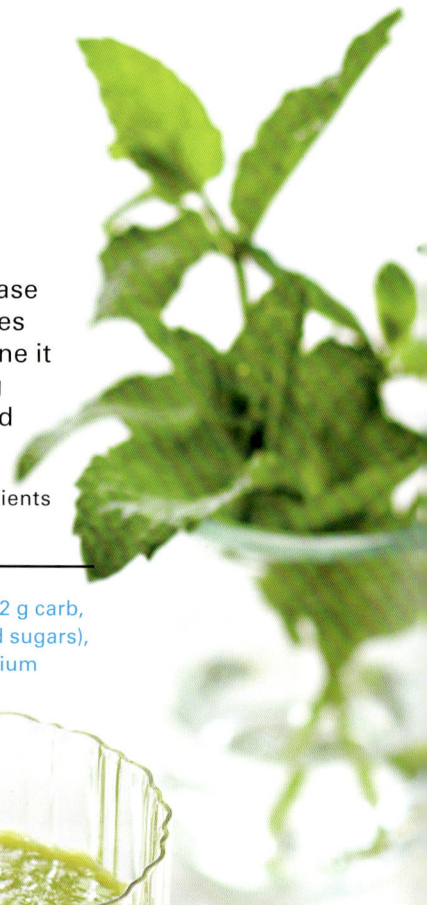

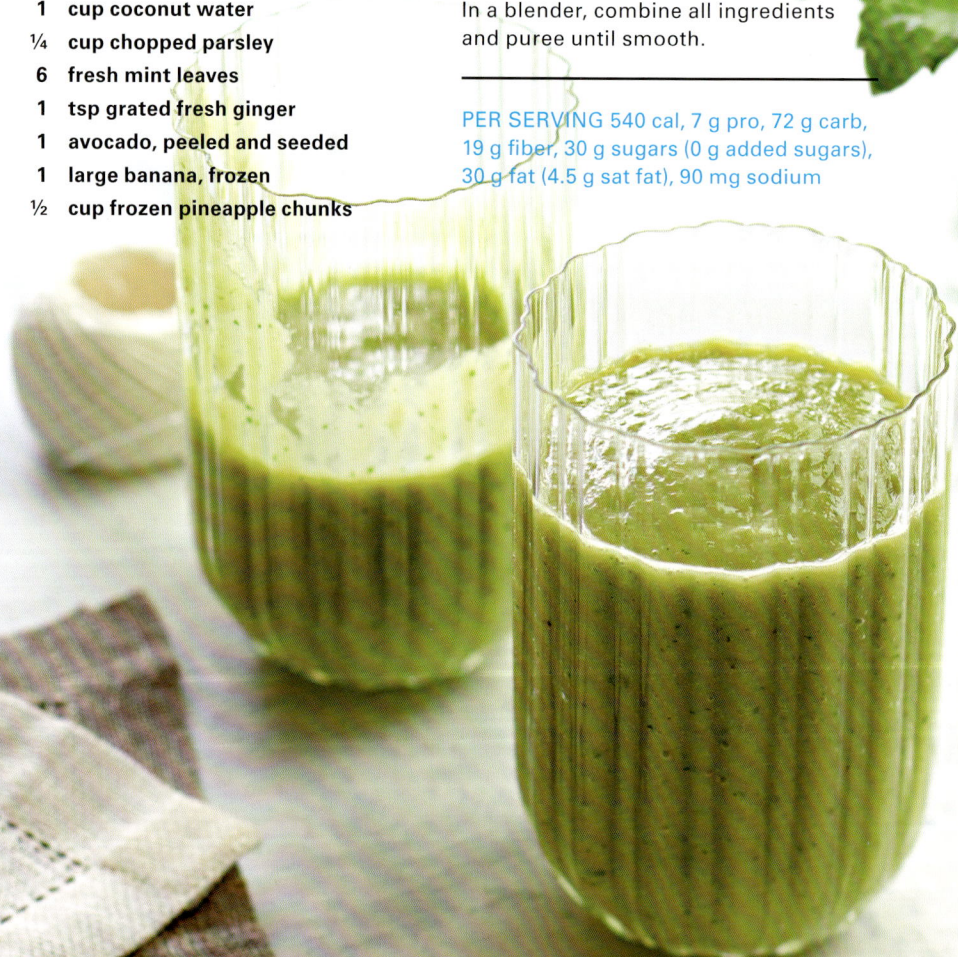

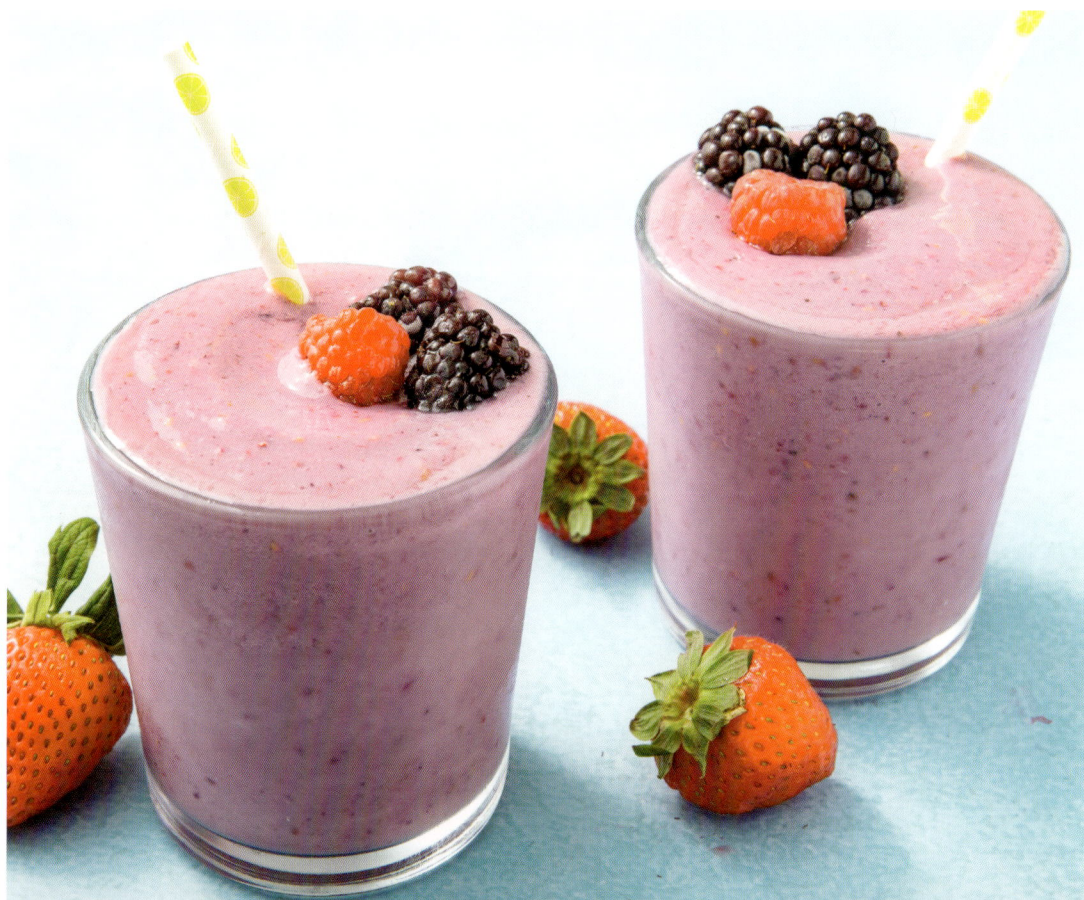

Triple Berry Smoothie

HIGH FIBER
PROTEIN-PACKED

TOTAL **5 MIN**. // SERVES **1**

This colorful smoothie tastes as good as it looks. You'll throw in banana and a mix of berries—strawberries, blackberries, and raspberries—along with almond milk and Greek yogurt for an energizing mix of protein and nutrients.

⅔ **cup almond milk**

½ **cup Greek yogurt**

½ **banana**

½ **cup frozen strawberries**

½ **cup frozen blackberries, plus more for garnish (optional)**

½ **cup frozen raspberries**

In a blender, combine all ingredients and puree until smooth. Serve topped with additional blackberries, if desired.

PER SERVING
315 cal, 15 g pro, 47 g carb, 12 g fiber, 27 g sugars (0 g added sugars), 9 g fat (3.5 g sat fat), 170 mg sodium

Sunshine Daydream Smoothie

TOTAL **5 MIN.** // SERVES **1**

Sugary cravings standing in the way of your weight loss goals? Stone fruits are naturally sweet, but they also happen to be pretty low in calories. We sweetened this smoothie with a half cup of peaches and mixed in fiber-rich strawberries and protein-packed yogurt for a tall glass of pure bliss. Cravings crushed!

½	**cup coconut water**
1	**cup plain yogurt**
1	**cup frozen strawberries**
½	**cup frozen peaches**
1	**fresh strawberry, for garnish**

In a blender, combine all ingredients and puree until smooth. Garnish with a strawberry, if desired.

PER SERVING 250 cal, 10 g pro, 36 g carb, 4 g fiber, 28 g sugars (0 g added sugars), 8 g fat (5 g sat fat), 150 mg sodium

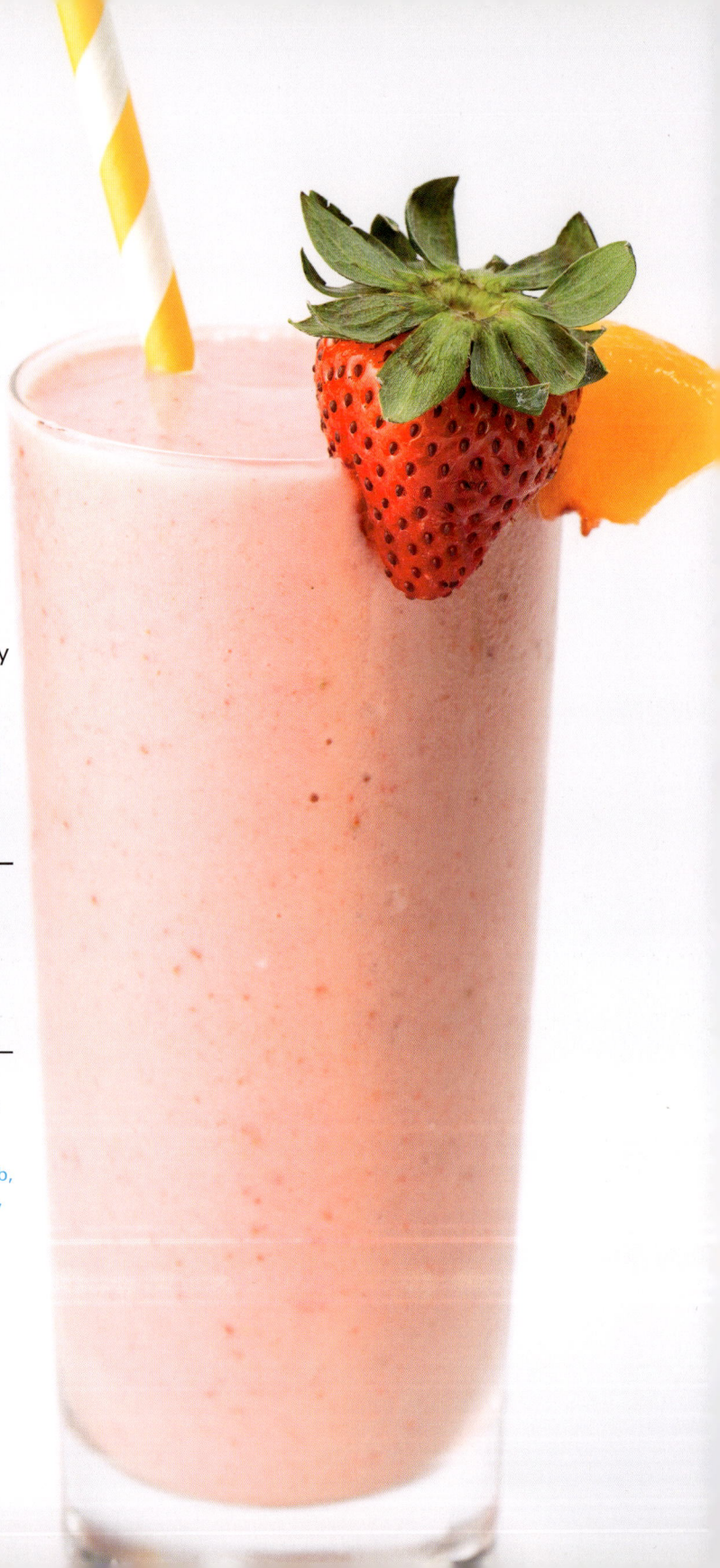

VEGAN **HIGH FIBER**

Strawberry-Watermelon Smoothie

TOTAL **5 MIN**. // SERVES **1**

The secret ingredient to this creamy smoothie? Potassium- and fiber-rich avocado— it's filling and satiating.

¼	cup almond milk
1	cup cubed watermelon
½	avocado
½	cup frozen strawberries

In a blender, combine all ingredients and puree until smooth.

PER SERVING 240 cal, 3 g pro, 29 g carb, 10 g fiber, 17 g sugars (0 g added sugars), 16 g fat (2 g sat fat), 60 g sodium

VEGAN **HIGH FIBER**

Blueberry Brain-Boost Smoothie

TOTAL **5 MIN**. // SERVES **1**

Blueberries help with digestive health, and the fruit has also been shown to improve cognitive function. Paired with walnuts, they make a blueberry smoothie that tops the antioxidant chart. And the rich nuttiness of the walnuts complements the berries so well, you'll love sipping this unforgettable smoothie!

½	cup apple juice
½	fresh ripe banana
2	Tbsp raw walnuts
¾	cup frozen blueberries
¼	cup frozen raspberries

In a blender, combine all ingredients and puree until smooth.

PER SERVING 295 cal, 4 g pro, 48 g carb, 8 g fiber, 31 g sugars (0 g added sugars), 11 g fat (1 g sat fat), 5 mg sodium

Pretty in Pink Raspberry Smoothie

TOTAL **5 MIN**. // SERVES **1**

Silken tofu adds a creamy texture and a hefty boost of protein to this hot pink smoothie recipe.

1	cup skim milk
½	cup orange juice
3	oz silken tofu
1½	cups frozen raspberries

In a blender, combine all ingredients and puree until smooth.

PER SERVING 290 cal, 16 g pro, 51 g carb, 14 g fiber, 32 g sugars (0 g added sugars), 4 g fat (0.5 g sat fat), 110 mg sodium

Banana-Blueberry Smoothie

TOTAL **5 MIN**. // SERVES **1**

This smoothie combines milk, ricotta cheese, and protein powder for the ultimate protein powerhouse, perfect for sipping after an intense sweat session.

¼	cup 1% milk
¾	cup ricotta cheese
2	tsp vanilla whey-protein powder
½	cup blueberries
½	banana
6	ice cubes

In a blender, combine all ingredients and puree until smooth.

PER SERVING 460 cal, 27 g pro, 33 g carb, 3 g fiber, 18 g sugars (0 g added sugars), 25.5 g fat (16 g sat fat), 195 mg sodium

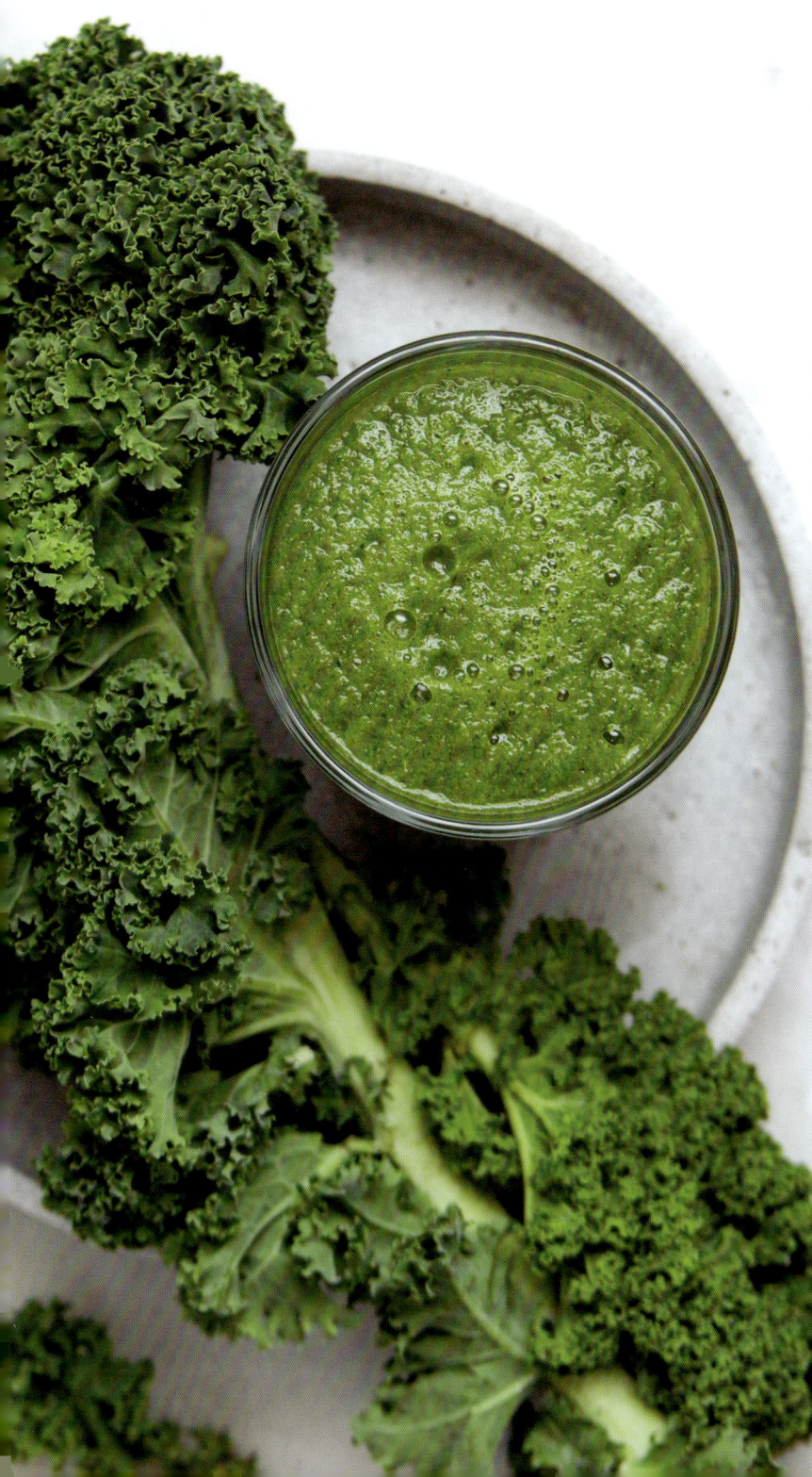

Kale Smoothie

TOTAL **5 MIN.** // SERVES **1**

Drinking a kale smoothie might sound horrible, but ours is actually delish. The sweetness of the banana and maple syrup offsets the bitterness of kale, while the almond milk keeps the calorie count low.

---

1   cup unsweetened almond milk

1   tsp maple syrup

1   Tbsp flaxseed

1   banana, sliced

¾   cup chopped kale (fresh or frozen)

1   cup ice

In a blender, combine all ingredients and puree until smooth.

PER SERVING 180 cal, 3 g pro, 35 g carb, 5 g fiber, 19 g sugars (4 g added sugars), 5 g fat (0.5 g sat fat), 190 mg sodium

Berry-Banana Smoothie

TOTAL **10 MIN.** // SERVES **1**

Resistant starch looks like a starch but acts like a fiber, passing through the small intestine to the colon without being digested. It's a starch that "resists" digestion. Oats add body to your smoothies, and the resistant starch this whole grain contains helps you feel fuller longer. An added bonus of resistant starch? It causes less gas than other fibers.

- 2 **Tbsp orange juice**
- ¼ **cup vanilla low-fat yogurt**
- 1 **tsp honey**
- ½ **banana, sliced**
- 2 **Tbsp rolled oats**
- ½ **cup frozen strawberries**

In a blender, combine all ingredients and puree until smooth.

PER SERVING 205 cal, 6 g pro, 45 g carb, 4 g fiber, 28 g sugars (11 g added sugars), 2 g fat (0.5 g sat fat), 45 mg sodium

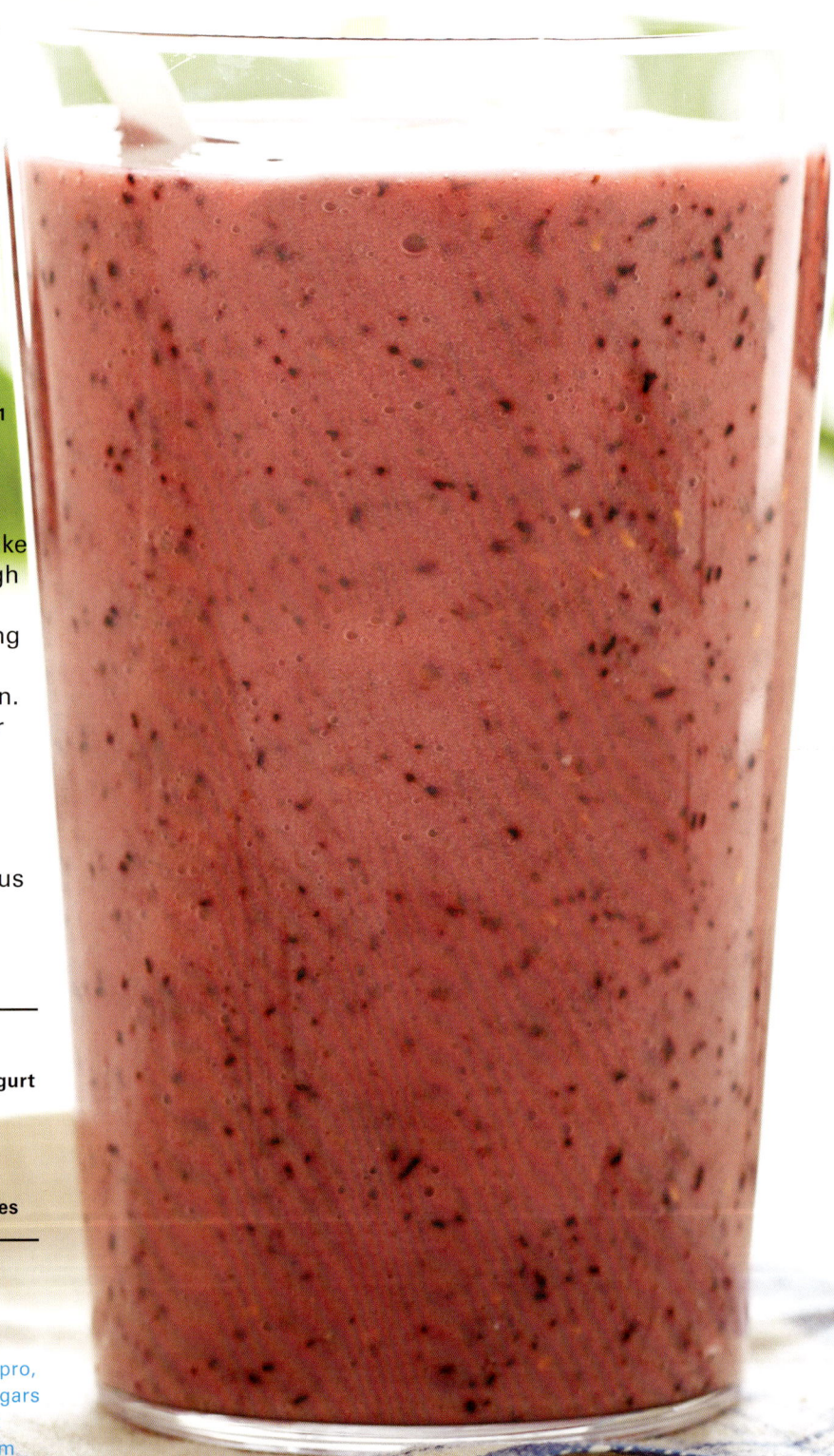

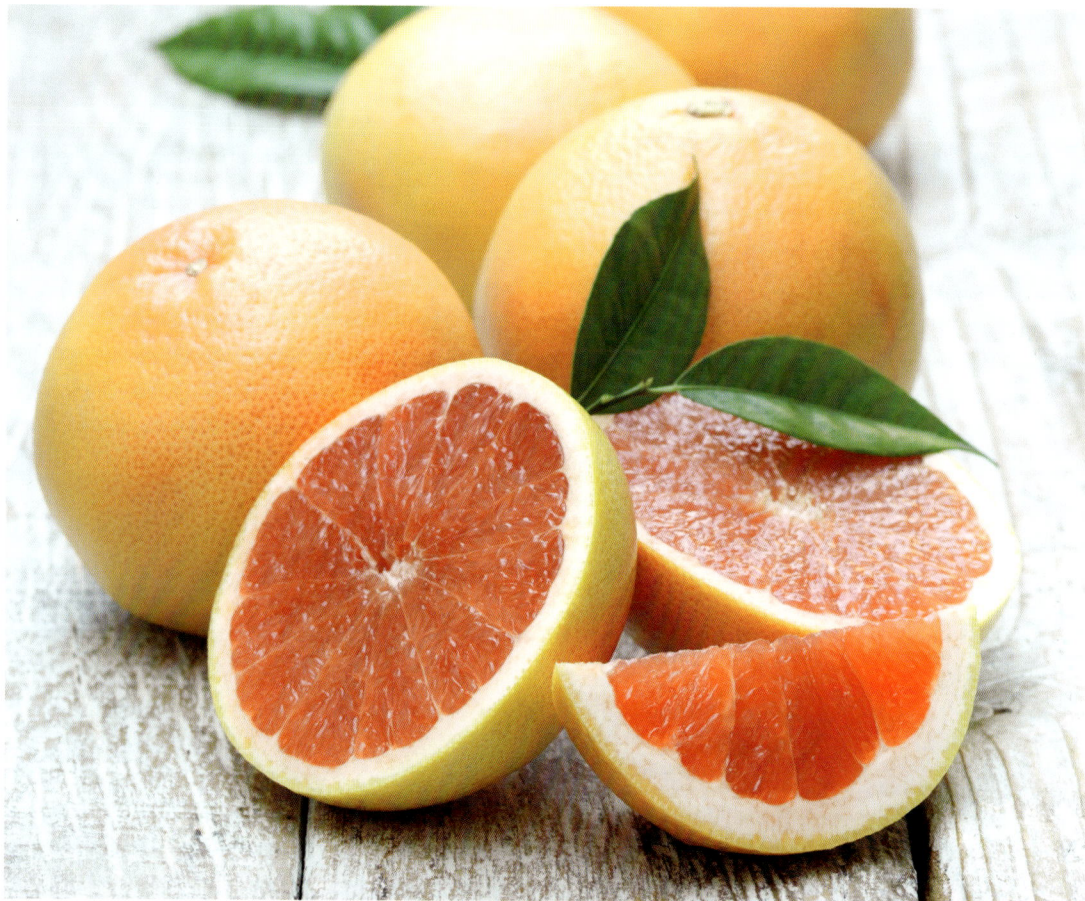

Grapefruit Banana Smoothie

VEGAN
HIGH FIBER

TOTAL **5 MIN.** // SERVES **1**

Grapefruit not only has a refreshing wake-me-up scent, it also has lots of water to keep you hydrated. Here, it's paired with bananas, which contain potassium, a mineral that helps your body with its daily functions. Blend up this sweet-tart combo for a strong start to your day.

1 cup unsweetened almond milk

1 pink grapefruit, peeled and segmented

1 frozen banana

½ cup frozen strawberries

In a blender, combine all ingredients and puree until smooth.

PER SERVING
275 cal, 5 g pro, 63 g carb, 9 g fiber, 41 g sugars (0 g added sugars), 4 g fat (0 g sat fat), 185 mg sodium

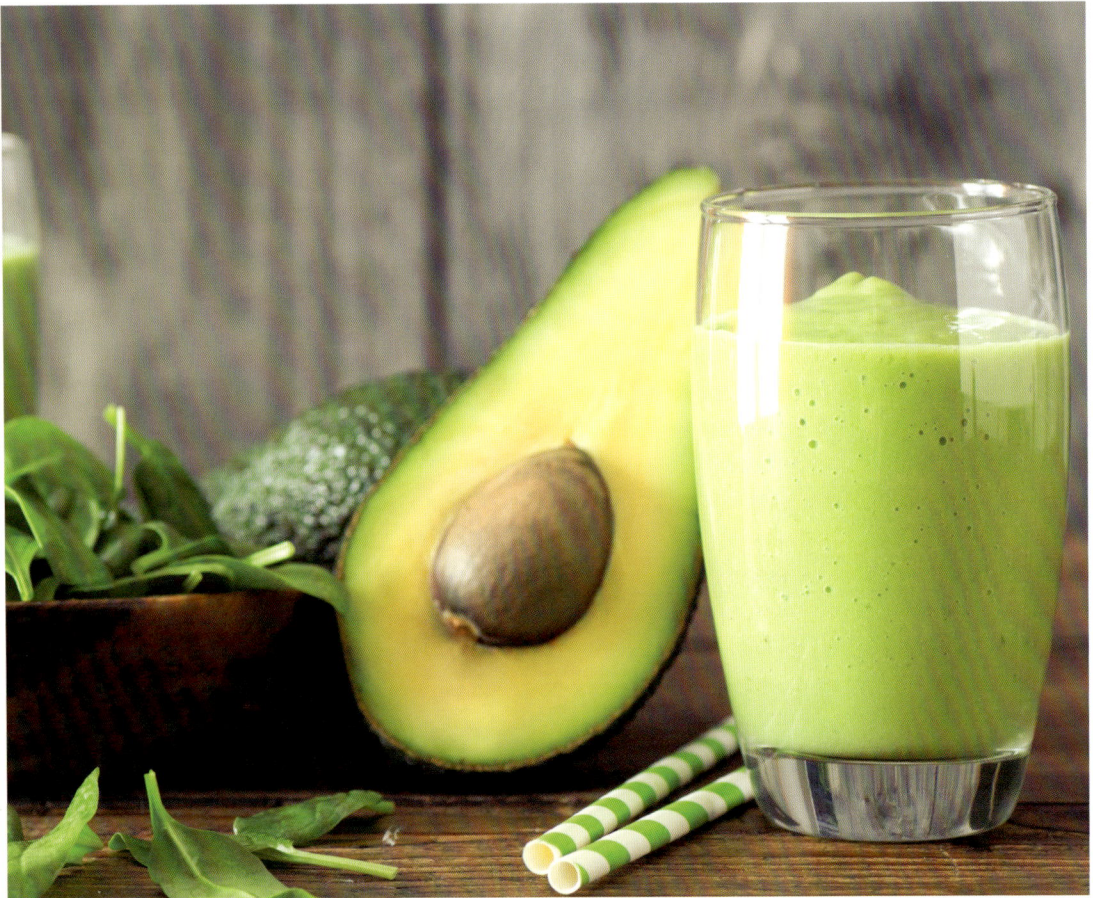

Berry, Orange & Avocado Smoothie

VEGAN
HIGH FIBER

TOTAL **5 MIN**. // SERVES **1**

This luscious smoothie gets a major green boost from tender baby spinach. And together, the ingredients offer a dose of potassium that adds up to 734 milligrams per serving, which is nearly 30% of your adequate intake (AI) for the day. Bottoms up!

- ⅔ **cup orange juice**
- ¼ **avocado, pitted and peeled**
- ½ **cup packed baby spinach**
- ½ **cup frozen mixed berries**
- ½ **cup ice cubes**

In a blender, combine all ingredients and puree until smooth.

PER SERVING
190 cal, 3 g pro,
30 g carb, 6 g fiber,
19 g sugars
(0 g added sugars),
7 g fat (1 g sat fat),
20 mg sodium

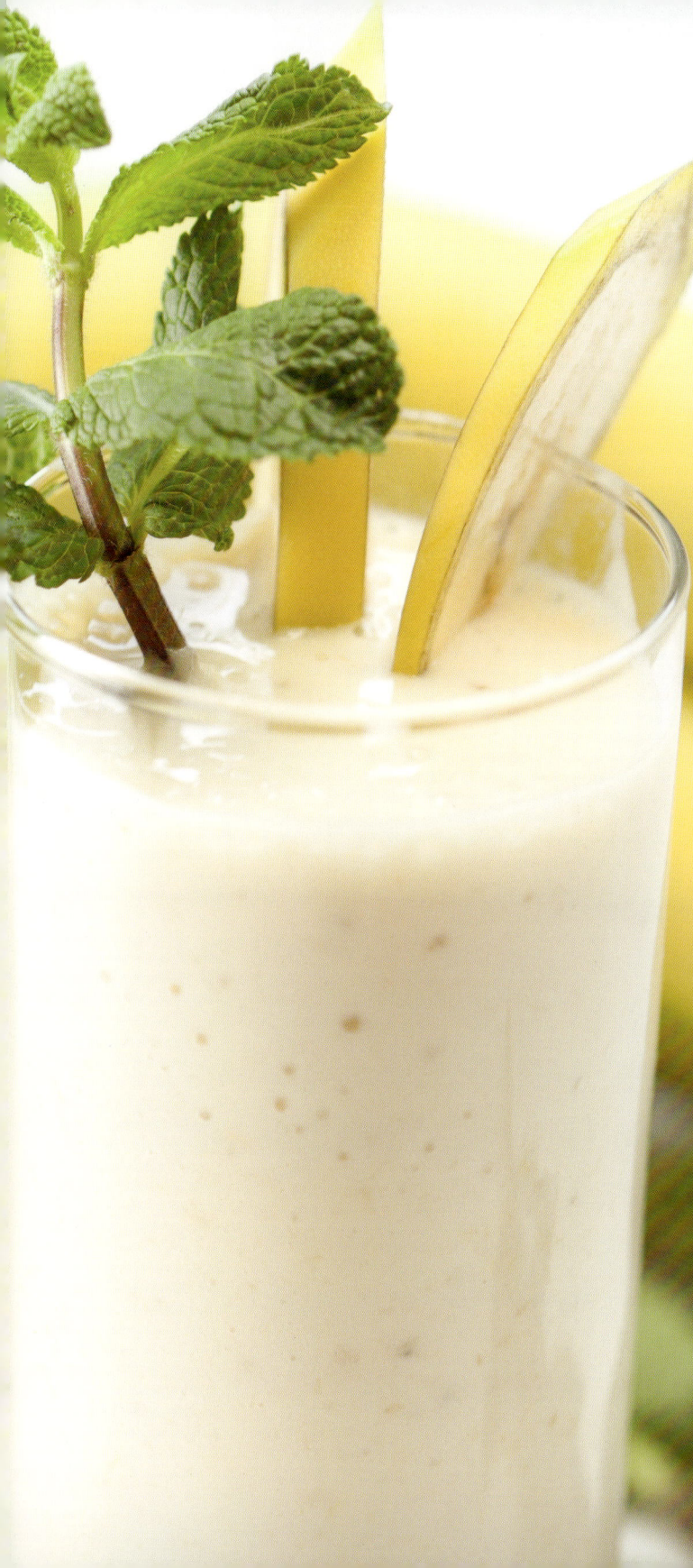

Potassium Peppermint Smoothie

TOTAL **5 MIN. PLUS SOAKING TIME**
SERVES **1**

Every tough workout deserves an equally great reward. Treat yourself with this minty smoothie, packed with muscle-building protein to help you repair, refuel, and re-energize.

---

1   cup plain organic soy milk
⅓   cup silken tofu
¼   tsp vanilla extract
¼   cup fresh mint leaves (soaked in water overnight)
1   small frozen banana, sliced
1   cup ice
      Chopped cashews and/or rolled oats, for garnish (optional)

In a blender, combine all ingredients and puree until smooth. Top with a sprinkle of chopped cashews and/or rolled oats, if desired.

PER SERVING 370 cal, 17 g pro, 37 g carb, 12 g fiber, 15 g sugars (0 g added sugar), 19 g fat (3 g sat fat), 80 mg sodium

Cherry-Almond Smoothie

TOTAL 5 MIN. // **SERVES 1**

This creamy, fruity blend contains ingredients that help ease joint and muscle pain. Tart cherry juice helps reduce inflammation. Almond butter and yogurt contain magnesium, which aid in relaxing tight muscles. And collagen powder contains amino acids that boost bone health. Drink up and stay unstoppable!

- ½ **cup tart cherry juice**
- 1 **cup 2% Greek yogurt**
- 2 **Tbsp almond butter**
- 1-2 **Tbsp collagen powder**
- ½ **cup frozen Bing cherries**

In a blender, combine all ingredients and puree until smooth.

PER SERVING 485 cal, 40 g pro, 44 g carb, 5 g fiber, 32 g sugars (0 g added sugars), 23 g fat (4 g sat fat), 120 mg sodium

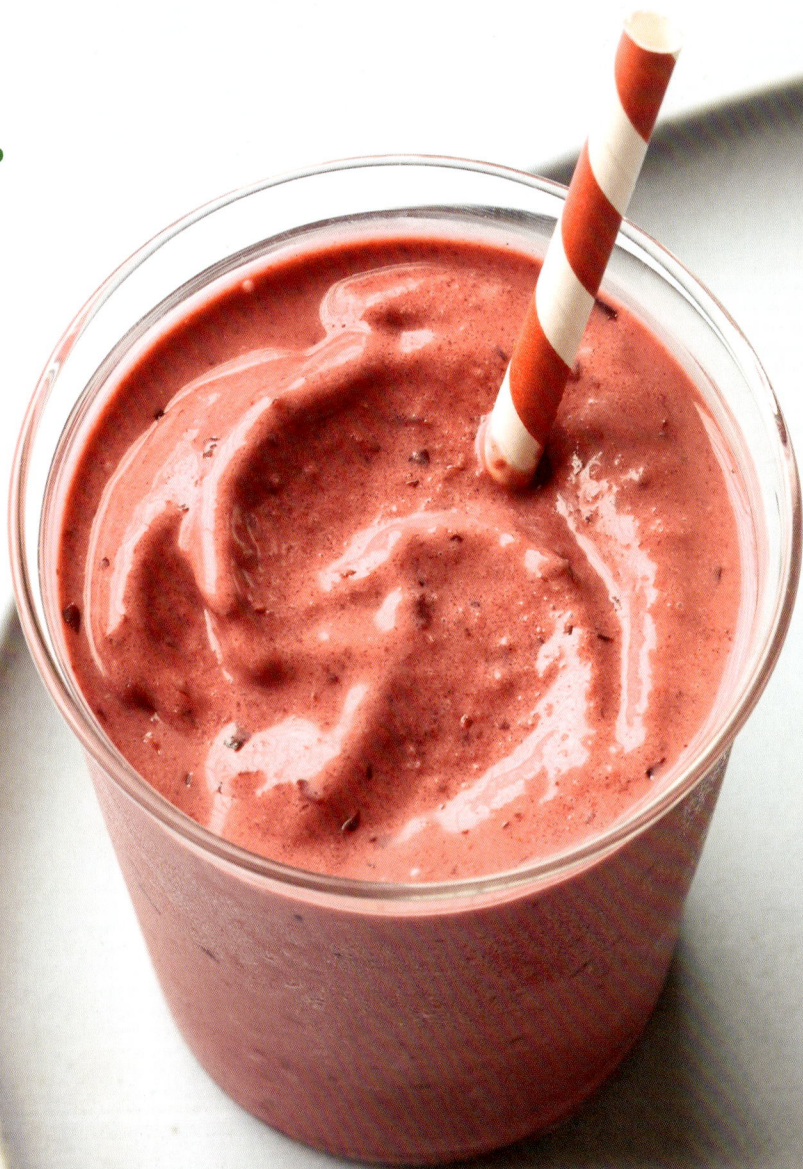

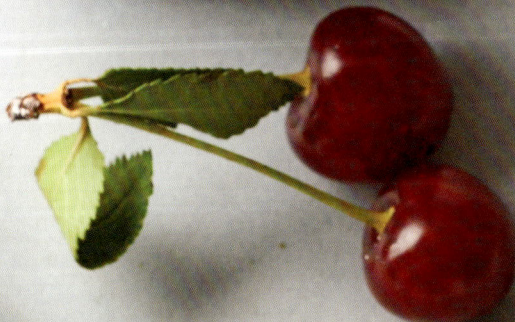

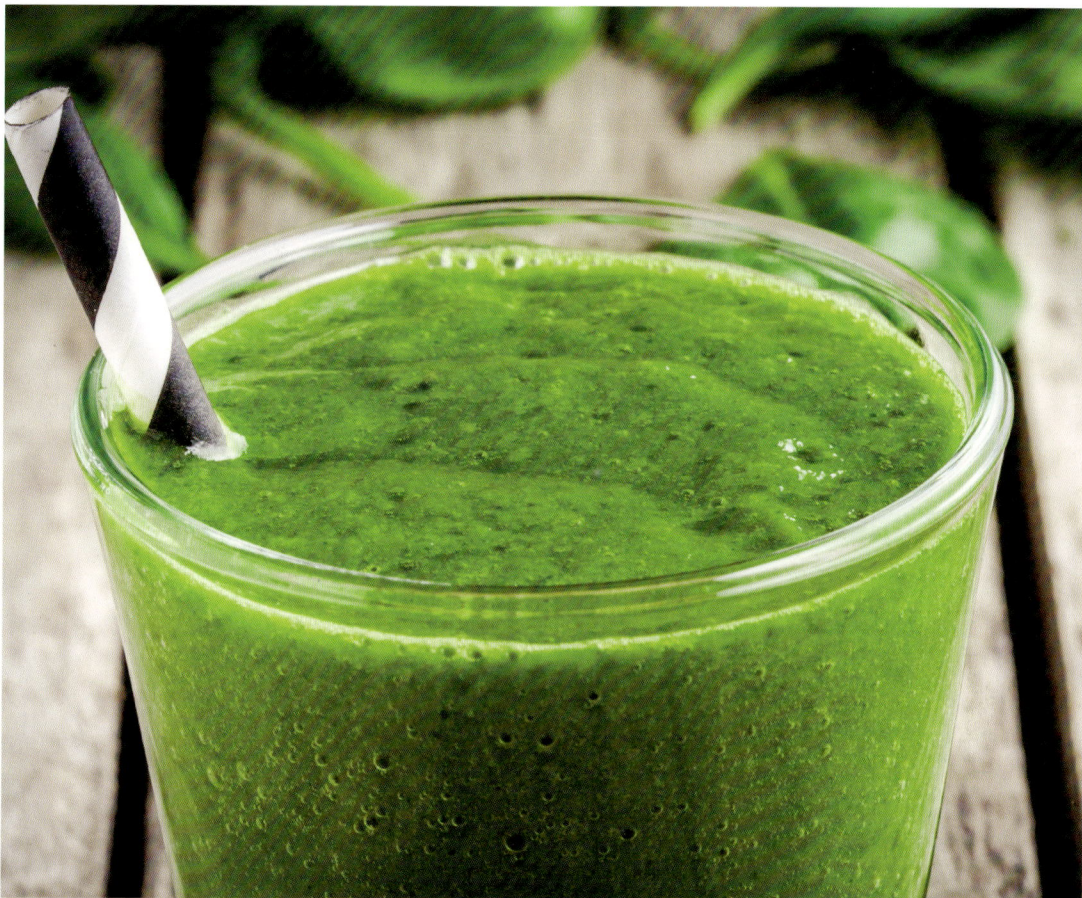

Green Apple Smoothie

TOTAL **5 MIN.** // SERVES **1**

VEGAN
PROTEIN-PACKED
HIGH FIBER

Athletes have higher iron needs than the average person because they lose more of this vital mineral through wear and tear, sweat, and through their GI system. When you're low in iron, you can't make enough red blood cells, leading to less oxygen being transported to your muscles. Help replenish your stores with this protein- and iron-packed sipper.

¾   **cup water**
½   **green apple, cored and chopped**
1   **cup baby spinach**
1   **Tbsp nut butter**
1   **scoop unsweetened whey protein powder**
    Handful of ice (optional)

In a blender, combine all ingredients and puree until smooth.

PER SERVING
230 cal, 21 g pro, 20 g carb, 5 g fiber, 11 g sugars (0 g added sugars), 10 g fat (2 g sat fat), 110 mg sodium

Peanut Butter Banana Smoothie

TOTAL **5 MIN**. // SERVES **1**

This smoothie recipe works overtime, blending sweet banana, creamy Greek yogurt, and natural smooth peanut butter for a good dose of muscle-building protein and filling fiber, all while satisfying your sweet tooth.

1	cup unsweetened almond milk
2	Tbsp peanut butter (preferably natural)
2	tsp honey
⅛	tsp pure vanilla extract
⅛	tsp ground cinnamon
2	small bananas or 1 large one
1	cup ice

In a blender, combine all ingredients and puree until smooth.

PER SERVING 475 cal, 11 g pro, 66 g carb, 9 g fiber, 37 g sugars (12 g added sugars), 20 g fat (3 g sat fat), 290 mg sodium

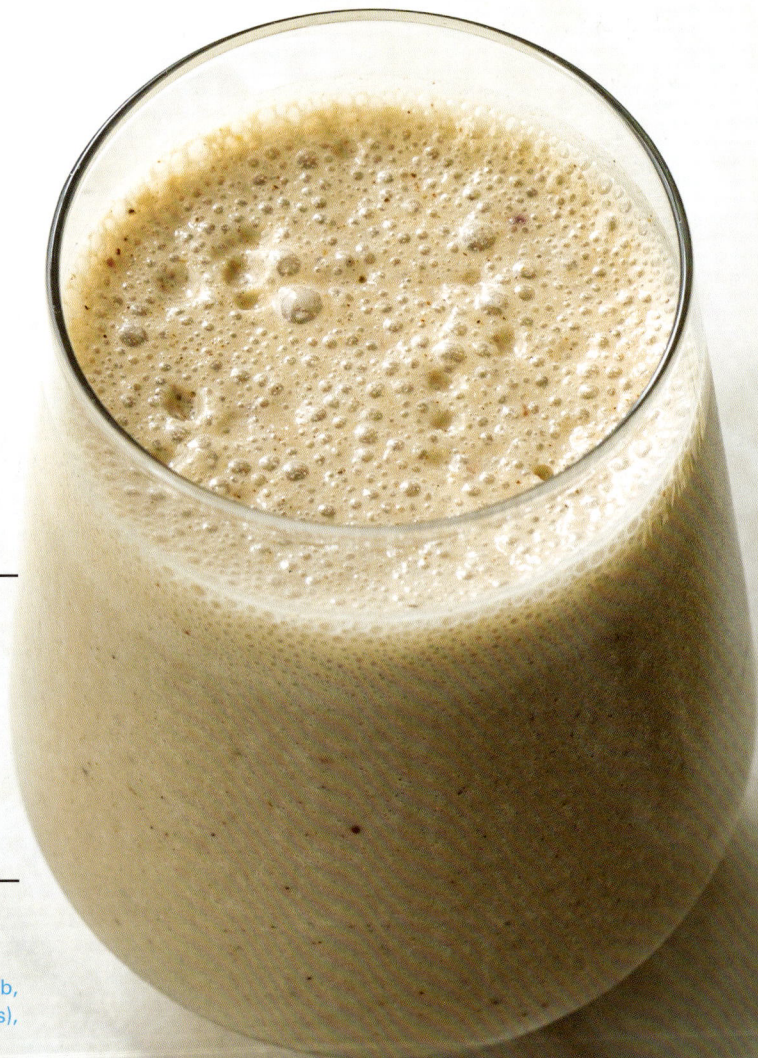

VEGAN HIGH FIBER PROTEIN-PACKED

Banana-Strawberry Breakfast Smoothie

TOTAL **5 MIN**. // SERVES **1**

This classic smoothie combination gets a protein boost, which makes for a satisfying early morning post-workout breakfast.

- ½   **cup cold orange juice**
- 1   **banana, sliced**
- ½   **scoop protein powder (preferably plant-based)**
- ¾   **cup frozen strawberries**

In a blender, combine all ingredients and puree until smooth.

PER SERVING 260 cal, 15 g pro, 51 g carb, 6 g fiber, 30 g sugars (0 g added sugars), 2 g fat (0.5 g sat fat), 170 mg sodium

Creamy Cantaloupe-Lime Smoothie

TOTAL **10 MIN**. // SERVES **1**

Cantaloupe is 90% water. Combine it with the muscle-building power of protein-packed yogurt, and you have the perfect smoothie to drink after your next sweat session.

- ½   **cup vanilla yogurt**
- ½   **tsp lime zest plus 1 Tbsp juice**
- 2   **cups diced cantaloupe**
- ½   **peach, chopped (about ⅓ cup)**
- ¼   **cup ice cubes**

In a blender, combine all ingredients and puree until smooth.

PER SERVING 265 cal, 9 g pro, 51 g carb, 4 g fiber, 46 g sugars (8 g added sugars), 5 g fat (2.5 g sat fat), 130 mg sodium

Green Pineapple Coconut Smoothie

TOTAL **10 MIN.** // SERVES **1**

Potassium is an essential mineral that protects you against annoyances like leg cramps and serious issues like stroke. Many adults don't get enough, though, so change that by starting your day with this tropical smoothie that packs a potassium punch with spinach and banana.

½	**cup light coconut milk**
½	**Tbsp lime juice**
½	**tsp grated lime zest**
1	**cup baby spinach**
½	**cup frozen pineapple chunks**
½	**banana, sliced and frozen**

In a blender, combine all ingredients and puree until smooth.

PER SERVING 190 cal, 4 g pro, 30 g carb, 4 g fiber, 11.5 g sugars (0 g added sugars), 7 g fat (7 g sat fat), 45 mg sodium

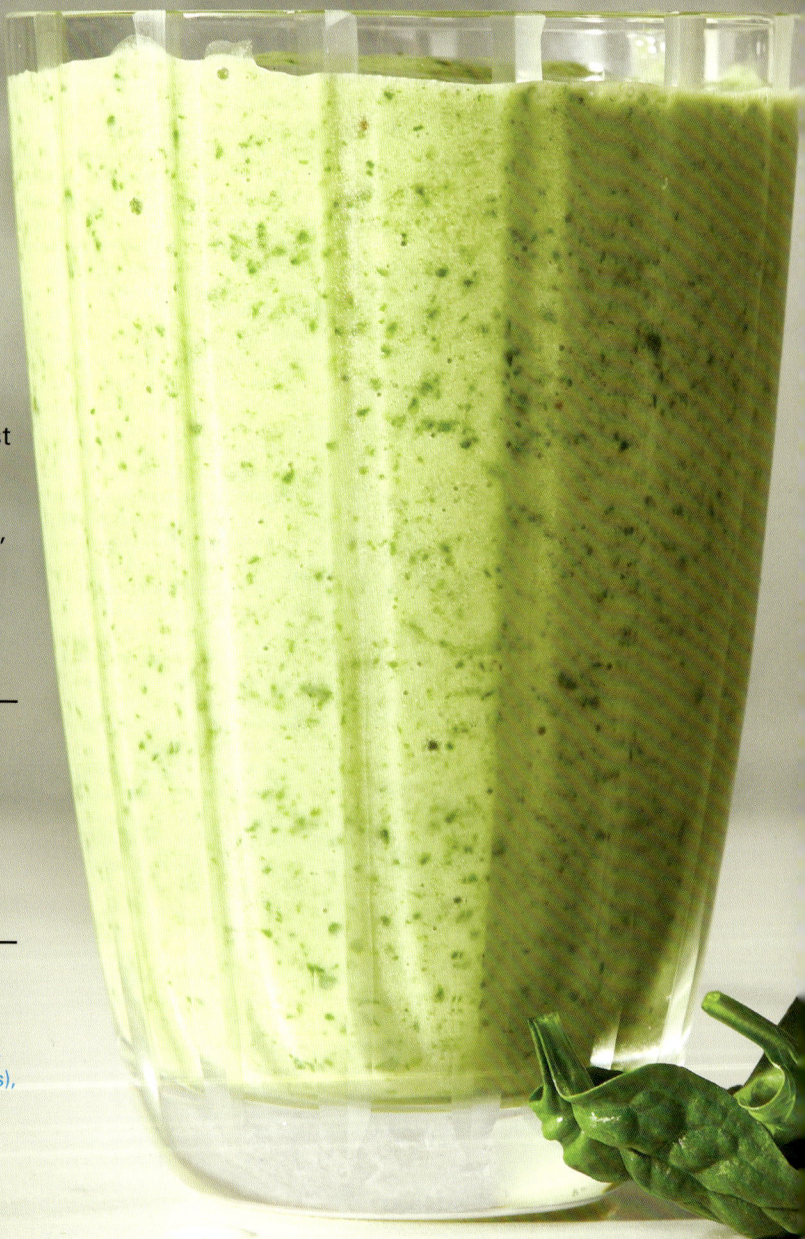

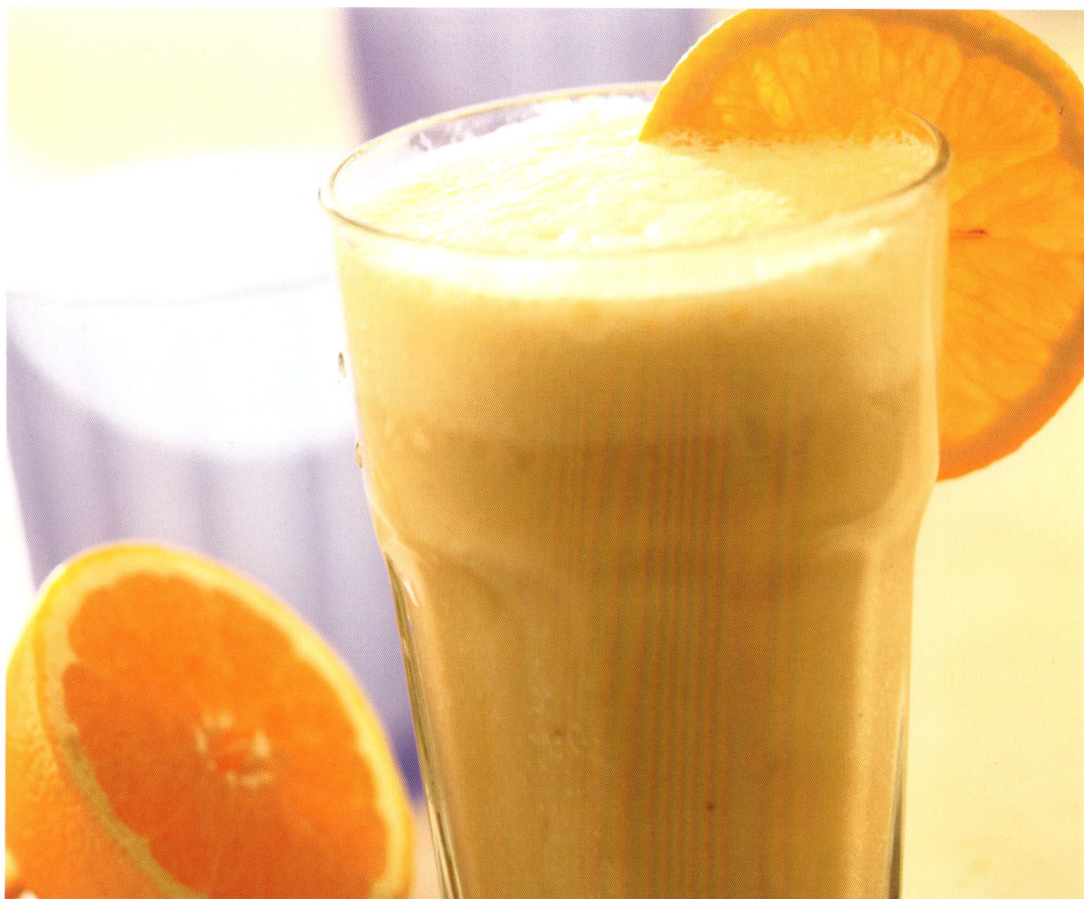

Orange Sunrise

VEGAN

TOTAL **5 MIN**. // SERVES **1**

Wake up to this refreshing smoothie recipe. The yogurt makes for a filling sip, while the bright orange juice and zest give this smoothie just the right amount of zing to start your day right. Pair it with a hard-boiled egg or almond butter toast if you're looking to make it a more substantial meal to get you through the morning.

1	cup vanilla soy milk
½	cup cold orange juice
1	tsp orange zest
¼	cup ice cubes

In a blender, combine all ingredients and puree until smooth.

PER SERVING
165 cal, 7 g pro, 25 g carb, 1 g fiber, 19 g sugars (8 g added sugars), 4 g fat (0.5 g sat fat), 115 mg sodium

Gut-Friendly Smoothie

TOTAL **5 MIN.** // SERVES **1**

We humans have a long history of eating bananas: They're believed to have been grown as an edible crop since at least 300 B.C.E.! In addition to fiber, bananas also contain inulin, a prebiotic that supports digestive health. Drink up for a happy gut!

---

1   cup almond milk
3   Tbsp chocolate protein powder
3   Tbsp peanut butter powder
1   ripe banana
1   shot espresso for flavor, optional
1   Tbsp flaxseed meal, optional

In a blender, combine all ingredients and puree until smooth.

PER SERVING 355 cal, 26 g pro, 47 g carb, 7 g fiber, 19 g sugars (2 g added sugars), 8 g fat (1 g sat fat), 570 mg sodium

TIP
If you don't have protein and peanut powders, substitute ½ cup Greek yogurt, ½ cup of any kind of milk, and 1 Tbsp peanut butter; add banana and blend.

Credits

This book is intended as a reference volume only, not as a medical manual. The information given here is designed to help you make informed decisions about your health. It is not intended as a substitute for any treatment that may have been prescribed by your doctor. If you suspect that you have a medical problem, we urge you to seek competent medical help.

Mention of specific companies, organizations, or authorities in this book does not imply endorsement by the author or publisher, nor does mention of specific companies, organizations, or authorities imply that they endorse this book, its author, or the publisher.

Internet addresses and telephone numbers given in this book were accurate at the time it went to press.

COVER PHOTOGRAPH by Evi Abeler
COVER FOOD STYLING by Simon Andrews
BOOK DESIGN by Gillian MacLeod

Library of Congress Cataloging-in-Publication Data is on file with the publisher.

ISBN 978-1-955710-02-2

2 4 6 8 10 9 7 5 3 paperback

Printed in China

HEARST

INTERIOR PHOTOGRAPHY

alpaksoy/iStock/Getty Images Plus: 170; Laurie Ambrose/Moment/Getty Images: 118 (bottom left); Amguy/iStock/Getty Images Plus: 65; Verdina Anna/Moment/Getty Images: 10; Arx0nt/iStock/Getty Images Plus: 71, 138; Arx0nt/Moment/Getty Images: 126; James Baigrie: 77; Aksana Ban/Moment/Getty Images: 123; Ethan Calabrese: 145, 154, 160; carlosgaw/E+/Getty Images: 118 (top left); cegli/iStock/Getty Images Plus: 72; Chris Court: 98; Adrian Crook/Moment/Getty Images: 118 (bottom right); c_yung/iStock/Getty Images Plus: 167; Danielle Daly: 80, 88, 108, 112, 172; Parker Feierbach: 159; Philip Friedman: 94; fudfoto/iStock/Getty Images Plus: 75; Mike Garten: 79, 82, 86, 90-92, 100, 106, 110, 114-116, 132, 134, 136–137, 146, 153, 174; Alison Gootee: 149; Brian Hagiwara/The Image Bank/Getty Images: 118 (top right); intek1/iStock/Getty Images Plus: 128; IriGri8/iStock/Getty Images Plus: 141; izhairguns/E+/Getty Images: 163; Johner Images/Getty Images: 157; Kang Kim: 117; Lauren King/EyeEm/Getty Images: 122; Martina Lanotte/EyeEm/Getty Images: 129; larik_malasha/iStock/Getty Images Plus: 102; Lecic/iStock/Getty Images Plus: 150, 166; LightFieldStudios/iStock/Getty Images Plus: 140; LindasPhotography/iStock/Getty Images Plus: 22 (bottom right); David Malosh: 64, 69-70, 73, 168; Mitch Mandel: 142–143, 173; Kate Mathis: 164; Diana Miller/Image Source/Getty Images: 131, 165; Moyo Studio/E+/Getty Images: 15; Marija Neuwirth/EyeEm/Getty Images: 130; Vladislav Nosick/500px Plus/Getty Images: 125; olgaperepelova/Adobe Stock Images: 139; Con Poulos: 104; Linda Pugliese: 63, 67, 76; Anna Pustynnikova/iStock/Getty Images Plus: 68, 127; Ralucahphotography.ro/Moment/Getty Images: 22 (top); Lucy Schaeffer: 133; Science Photo Library/Getty Images: 22 (bottom left); Christopher Testani: 84, 96; Claudia Totir/Moment/Getty Images: 124; tvirbickis/iStock/Getty Images Plus: 62; Westend61/Getty Images: 66, 74; wmaster890/iStock/Getty Images Plus: 169; Oscar Wong/Moment/Getty Images: 9, 16-17; YBoiko/iStock/Getty Images Plus: 135

RECIPE DEVELOPMENT

The Delish Test Kitchen: 154, 161 (right); The Good Housekeeping Test Kitchen: 77-83, 89-91, 109-115, 134, 136–144, 147, 152 (right)–153, 155–156 (left), 157–158, 164, 171, 173; The Prevention Test Kitchen: 62-65, 67-76, 87, 93, 99-101, 105, 117, 135, 149, 151, 166-169, 172; Liza de Fazio: 165; Lindsay Funston: 145, 160; Makinze Gore: 159; Laura Russell Griffin: 150; Men's Health: 162 (right); Lindsay Maitland Hunt: 148 (right), 163, 170; Khalil Hymore: 85, 97; Aya Kanai: 162 (left); Joyann King: 161 (left); Frances Largeman-Roth, R.D.N.: 122–131; Jessica Matthews, M.S.: 66; Kate Merker: 107, 116; Arrica Elin Sansome: 132 (shared by Devin Miles), 133 (shared by Lorinda Sorensen, N.D.), 148 (left, shared by Carrie Baldwin-Sayre, N.D.), 152 (left, shared by Caitlin Policastro, N.P.), 174 (shared by Bronwyn Carlblom, N.M.D.); Margaret Yannucci: 156 (right)

THANK YOU FOR PURCHASING
The Smoothie Plan

Visit our online store to find more great products
from Prevention and save 20% off your next purchase.

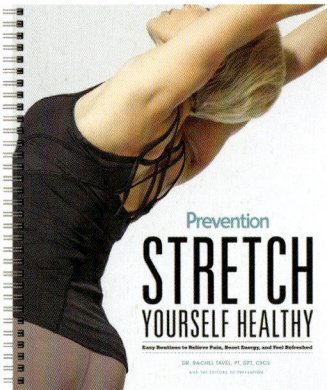

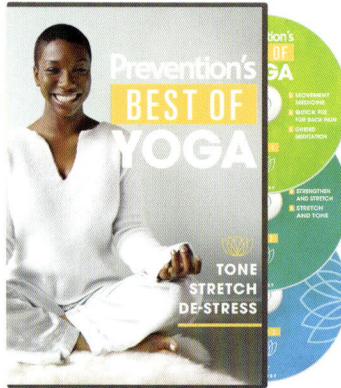

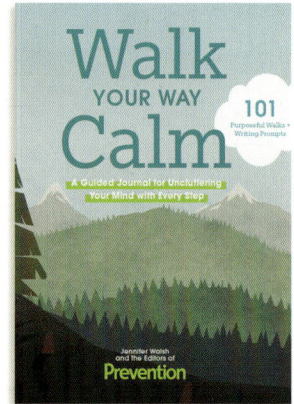